STATISTICS AT SQUARE TWO

STATISTICS AT SQUARE TWO:
Understanding modern statistical applications in medicine

M J Campbell
Professor of Medical Statistics
University of Sheffield, Sheffield

First published in 2001
Second impression 2002
by the BMJ Publishing Group, BMA House, Tavistock Square,
London WC1H 9JR
www.bmjbooks.com

British Library Cataloguing in Publication Data

A catalogue record for this book is available from the British Library

ISBN 0-7279-1394-8

Cover design by Egelnick & Webb, London
Typeset by FiSH Books, London
Printed and bound by J. W. Arrowsmith Ltd., Bristol

Contents

CONTENTS

Preface

When *Statistics at Square One* was first published in 1976 the type of statistics seen in the medical literature was relatively simple: means and medians, *t* tests and chi-squared tests. Carrying out complicated analyses then required arcane skills in calculation and computers, and was restricted to a minority who had undergone considerable training in data analysis. Since then, statistical methodology has advanced considerably and, more recently, statistical software has become available to enable research workers to carry out complex analyses with little effort. It is now commonplace to see advanced statistical methods used in medical research, but often the training received by the practitioners has been restricted to a cursory reading of a software manual. I have this nightmare of investigators actually learning statistics by reading a computer package manual. This means that much statistical methodology is used rather uncritically, and the data to check whether the methods are valid are often not provided when the investigators write up their results.

This book is intended to build on *Statistics at Square One*. It is hoped to be a "vade mecum" for investigators who have undergone a basic statistics course, to extend and explain what is found in the statistical package manuals and help in the presentation and reading of the literature. It is also intended for readers and users of the medical literature, but is intended to be rather more than a simple "bluffer's guide". Hopefully it will encourage the user to seek professional help when necessary. Important sections in each chapter are tips on reporting about a particular technique and the book emphasises correct interpretation of results in the literature.

Since most researchers do not want to become statisticians, detailed explanations of the methodology will be avoided. I hope it will prove useful to students on postgraduate courses and for this reason there are a number of exercises.

The choice of topics reflects what I feel are commonly

encountered in the medical literature, based on many years of statistical refereeing. The linking theme is regression models, and we cover multiple regression, logistic regression, Cox regression, Ordinal regression and Poisson regression. The predominant philosophy is frequentist, since this reflects the literature and what is available in most packages. However, a section on the uses of Bayesian methods is given.

Probably the most important contribution of statistics to medical research is in the design of studies. I make no apology for an absence of direct design issues here, partly because I think an investigator should consult a specialist to design a study and partly because there are a number of books available: Cox (1966), Altman (1991), Armitage and Berry (1995), Campbell and Machin (1999).

Most of the concepts in statistical inference have been covered in *Statistics at Square One*. In order to keep this book short, reference will be made to the earlier book for basic concepts. All the analyses described here have been conducted in STATA6 (STATACorp, 1999). However most, if not all, can also be carried out using common statistical packages such as SPSS, SAS, StatDirect or Splus. I am grateful to Stephen Walters and Mark Mullee for comments on various chapters and particularly to David Machin and Ben Armstrong for detailed comments on the manuscript. Further errors are my own.

MJ Campbell
Sheffield

Further reading

Armitage P, Berry G. *Statistical Methods in Medical Research.* Oxford: Blackwell Scientific publications, 1995.

Altman DG. *Practical Statistics in Medical Research.* London: Chapman and Hall, 1991.

Campbell MJ, Machin D. *Medical Statistics: a commonsense approach, 3rd edn.* Chichester: John Wiley, 1999.

Cox DR. *Planning of Experiments.* New York: John Wiley, 1966.

Swinscow TDV. *Statistics at Square One, 9th edn.* (revised by MJ Campbell). London: BMJ Books, 1996.

STATACorp. STATA Statistical Software Release 6.0. College Station, TX: STATA Corporation, 1999.

1 Models, tests and data

Summary

This chapter introduces the idea of a *statistical model* and then links it to *statistical tests*. The use of statistical models greatly expands the utility of statistical analysis. The different types of *data* that commonly occur in medical research are described, because knowing how the data arise will help one to choose a particular statistical model.

1.1 Basics

Much medical research can be simplified as an investigation of an input/output relationship. The inputs, or explanatory variables, are thought to be related to the outcome, or *effect*. We wish to investigate whether one or more of the input variables are plausibly causally related to the effect. The relationship is complicated by other factors that are thought to be related to both the cause and the effect; these are *confounding factors*. A simple example would be the relationship between stress and high blood pressure. Does stress cause high blood pressure? Here the causal variable is a measure of stress, which we assume can be quantified, and the outcome is a blood pressure measurement. A confounding factor might be gender; men may be more prone to stress, but they may also be more prone to high blood pressure. If gender is a confounding factor, a study would need to take gender into account.

An important start in the analysis of data is to determine which variables are inputs, and of these which do we wish to investigate as causal, which variables are outputs and which are confounders. Of course, depending on the question, a variable might serve as any of these. In a survey of the effects of smoking on chronic bronchitis, smoking is a causal variable. In a clinical trial to examine the effects of cognitive behavioural therapy on smoking habit, smoking is an outcome. In the above study of stress and high blood pressure, smoking may be a confounder.

However, before any analysis is done, and preferably in the original protocol, the investigator should decide on the causal, outcome and confounder variables.

1.2 Models

The relationship between inputs and outputs can be described by a mathematical model which relates the inputs, both causal variables and confounders (often called "independent variables" and denoted by x) with the output (often called the dependent variable and denoted by y). Thus in the stress and blood pressure example above, we denote blood pressure by y and stress and gender are both x variables. We wish to know if stress is still a good predictor of blood pressure when we know an individual's gender. To do this we need to assume that gender and stress combine in some way to affect blood pressure. As discussed in Swinscow,[1] we describe the models at a *population* level. We take samples to get estimates of the population values. In general we will refer to population values using Greek letters, and estimates using Roman letters.

The most commonly used models are known as "linear models". They assume that the x variables combine in a linear fashion to predict y. Thus if x_1 and x_2 are the two independent variables we assume that an equation of the form $\beta_0 + \beta_1 x_1 + \beta_2 x_2$ is the best predictor of y where β_0, β_1 and β_2 are constants and are known as *parameters* of the model. The method often used for estimating the parameters is known as *regression* and so these are the *regression parameters*. Of course, no model can predict the y variable perfectly, and the model acknowledges this by incorporating an *error* term. These linear models are appropriate when the outcome variable is Normally distributed.[1] The wonderful aspect of these models is that they can be generalised so that the modelling procedure is similar for many different situations, such as when the outcome is non-Normal or discrete. Thus different areas of statistics, such as t tests and chi-squared tests are unified, and dealt with in a similar manner using a method known as "generalised linear models".

When we have taken a sample, we can estimate the parameters of the model, and get a fit to the data. A simple description of the way that data relate to the model[2] is

$$DATA = FIT + RESIDUAL$$

The FIT is what is obtained from the model given the predictor variables. The RESIDUAL is the difference between the DATA and the FIT. For the linear model the residual is an estimate of the error term. For a generalised linear model this is not strictly the case, but the residual is useful for diagnosing poor fitting models as we shall see later.

Do not forget however, that models are simply an approximation to reality. "All models are wrong, but some are useful."

The subsequent chapters describe different models where the dependent variable takes different forms: continuous, binary, a survival time, and when the values are correlated in time. The rest of this chapter is a quick review of the basics covered in *Statistics at Square One*.

1.3 Types of data

Data can be divided into two main types: quantitative and qualitative. *Quantitative data* tends to be either continuous variables that one can measure, such as height, weight or blood pressure, or discrete such as numbers of children per family, or numbers of attacks of asthma per child per month. Thus count data are discrete and quantitative. Continuous variables are often described as having a Normal distribution, or being non-Normal. Having a Normal distribution means that if you plotted a histogram of the data it would follow a particular "bell-shaped" curve. In practice, provided the data cluster about a single central point, and the distribution is symmetric about this point, it would commonly be considered close enough to Normal for most tests requiring Normality to be valid. Here one would expect the mean and median to be close. Non-Normal distributions tend to have asymmetric distributions (skewed) and the means and medians differ. Examples of non-Normally distributed variables include age and salaries in a population. Sometimes the asymmetry is caused by outlying points that are in fact errors in the data and these need to be examined with care.

Note it is a misnomer to talk of "non-parametric" data instead of "non-Normally distributed" data. Parameters belong to models, and what is meant by "non-parametric" data is data to which we cannot apply models, although as we shall see later, this is often a too limited view of statistical methods! An important feature of quantitative data is that you can deal with the numbers as having real meaning, so for example you can take averages of the data. This is in contrast to qualitative data, where the numbers are often convenient labels.

Qualitative data tend to be categories, thus people are male or female, European, American or Japanese, they have a disease or are in good health. They can be described as *nominal* or *categorical*. If there are only two categories they are described as *binary* data. Sometimes the categories can be ordered, so for example a person can "get better", "stay the same," or "get worse". These are *ordinal* data. Often these will be scored, say, 1, 2, 3, but if you had two patients, one of whom got better and one of whom got worse, it makes no sense to say that on average they stayed the same! (A statistician is someone with their head in the oven and their feet in the fridge, but on average they are comfortable!) The important feature about ordinal data is that they can be ordered, but there is no obvious weighting system. For example it is unclear how to weight "healthy", "ill", or "dead" as outcomes. (Often, as we shall see later, either scoring by giving consecutive whole numbers to the ordered categories and treating the ordinal variable as a quantitative variable or dichomising the variable and treating it as binary may work well.) Count data, such as numbers of children per family appear ordinal, but here the important feature is that arithmetic is possible (2.4 children per family is meaningful). This is sometimes described as having *ratio* properties. A family with four children has twice as many children as one with two, but if we had an ordinal variable with four categories, say "strongly agree", "agree", "disagree", "strongly disagree", and scored them 1 to 4, we cannot say that "strongly disagree", scored 4, is twice "agree", scored 2!

Qualitative data can be formed by categorising continuous data. Thus blood pressure is a continuous variable, but it can be split into "normotension" or "hypertension". This often makes it easier to summarise, for example 10% of the population have hypertension is easier to comprehend than a statement giving the mean and standard deviation of blood pressure in the population, although from the latter one could deduce the former (and more besides).

When the dependent variable is continuous, we use multiple regression, described in Chapter 2. When it is binary we use logistic regression or survival analysis described in Chapters 3 and 4, respectively. If the dependent variable is ordinal we use ordinal regression described in Chapter 6 and if it is count data, we use Poisson regression, also described in Chapter 6. In general, the question about what type of data are the independent variables is less important.

1.4 Significance tests

Significance tests such as the chi-squared test and the t test and the interpretation of P values were described in *Statistics at Square One*.[1] The form of statistical significance testing is to set up a *null hypothesis*, and then collect data. Using the null hypothesis we test if the observed data are consistent with the null hypothesis. As an example, consider a clinical trial to compare a new diet with a standard to reduce weight in obese patients. The null hypothesis is that there is no difference between the two treatments in weight changes of the patients. The outcome is the difference in the mean weight after the two treatments. We can calculate the probability of getting the observed mean difference (or one more extreme) if the null hypothesis of no difference in the two diets were true. If this probability (the P value) is sufficiently small, we reject the null hypothesis and assume that the new diet differs from the standard. The usual method of doing this is to divide the mean difference in weight in the two diet groups by the estimated standard error of the difference and compare this ratio to either a t distribution (small sample) or a Normal distribution (large sample).

The test as described above is known as Student's t test, but the form of the test, whereby an estimate is divided by its standard error and compared to a Normal distribution is known as a *Wald test*.

There are, in fact, a large number of different types of statistical test. For Normally distributed data, they usually give the same P values, but for other types of data they can give different results. In the medical literature there are three different tests commonly used and it is important to be aware of the basis of their construction and their differences. These tests are known as the *Wald test*, the *score test* and the *likelihood ratio test*. For non-Normally distributed data they can give different P values although usually the results converge as the data set increases in size. The basis for these three tests is described in Appendix 2.

1.5 Confidence intervals

The problem with statistical tests is that the P value depends on the size of the data set. With a large enough data set, it would be almost always possible to prove that two treatments differed significantly, albeit by small amounts. It is important to present the results of an analysis with an estimate of the mean effect, and a measure of precision, such as a confidence interval.[3] To understand a confidence interval we need to consider the difference between a population and a sample. A population is a group to whom we make generalisations, such as patients with diabetes, or middle-aged men. Populations have *parameters* such as the mean HbA1c in diabetics, or the mean blood pressure in middle-aged men. Models are used to model populations and so the parameters in a model are population parameters. We take samples to get *estimates* for model parameters. We cannot expect the estimate of a model parameter to be exactly equal to the true model parameter, but as the sample gets larger we would expect the estimate to get closer to the true value, and a confidence interval about the estimate helps to quantify this. A 95% confidence interval for a population mean implies that if we took one hundred samples of a fixed size, and calculated the mean and 95% confidence interval for each, then we would expect 95 of the intervals to include the true model parameter. The way they are commonly understood, from a single sample is that there is a 95% chance that the population parameter is in the 95% interval.

In the diet example given above, the confidence interval will measure how precisely we can estimate the effect of the new diet. If in fact the new diet were no different from the old, we would expect the confidence interval to contain zero.

1.6 Statistical tests using models

A t test compares the mean values of a continuous variable in two groups. This can be written as a linear model. In the example above, weight after treatment was the continuous variable, under one of two diets. Here the primary predictor variable x is diet, which is a binary variable taking the value (say) 0 for standard diet and 1 for the new diet. The outcome variable is weight. There are no confounding variables. The fitted model is

$$\text{Weight} = b_0 + b_1 \text{ diet} + \text{residual.}$$

The FIT part of the model is $b_0 + b_1$ diet and is what we would predict someone's weight to be given our estimate of the effect of the diet. We assume that the residuals have an approximate Normal distribution. The null hypothesis is that the coefficient associated with diet, b_1, is from a population with mean zero. Thus we assume that β_1, the population parameter, is zero.

Models enable us to make our assumptions explicit. A nice feature about models, as opposed to tests, is that they are easily extended. Thus, weight at baseline may (by chance) differ in the two groups, and will be related to weight after treatment, so it could be included as a confounder variable.

This method is further described in Chapter 2 using multiple regression. The treatment of the chi-squared test as a model is described in Chapter 3 under logistic regression.

1.7 Model fitting and analysis: exploratory and confirmatory analyses

There are two aspects to data analysis: confirmatory and exploratory analysis. In a *confirmatory analysis* we are testing a pre-specified hypothesis and it follows naturally to conduct significance tests. Testing for a treatment effect in a clinical trial is a good example of a confirmatory analysis. In an *exploratory analysis* we are looking to see what the data are telling us. An example would be looking for risk factors in a cohort study. The findings should be regarded as tentative to be confirmed in a subsequent study, and P values are largely decorative. Often one can do both types of analysis in the same study. For example, when analysing a clinical trial, a large number of possible outcomes may have been measured. Those specified in the protocol as primary outcomes are subjected to a confirmatory analysis, but there is often a large amount of information, say concerning side effects that could also be analysed. These should be reported, but with a warning that they emerged from the analysis and not from a pre-specified hypothesis. It seems illogical to ignore information in a study, but also the lure of an apparent unexpected significant result can be very difficult to resist (but should be)!

It may also be useful to distinguish *audit*, which is largely descriptive, intending to provide information about one particular time and place, and *research* which tries to be generalisable to other times and places.

1.8 Computer-intensive methods

Much of the theory described in the rest of this book requires some prescription of a distribution for the data, such as the Normal distribution. There are now methods available which use models but are less dependent on the actual distribution. They are very computer intensive and until recently were unfeasible. However they are becoming more prevalent, and for completeness a description of one such method, the *bootstrap* is given in Appendix 3.

1.9 Bayesian methods

The model based approach to statistics leads one to statements such as "given model M, the probability of obtaining data D is P". This is known as the *frequentist* approach. This assumes that population parameters are fixed. However, many investigators would like to make statements about the probability of model M being true, in the form "given the data D, what is the probability that model M is the correct one?" Thus one would like to know, for example, what is the probability of a diet working. A statement of this form would be particularly helpful for people who have to make decisions about individual patients. This leads to a way of thinking known as "Bayesian" and this allows population parameters to vary. This book is largely based on the frequentist approach. Most computer packages are also based on this approach. Further discussion is given in Chapter 5 and Appendix 4.

1.10 Reporting statistical results in the literature

The reporting of statistical results in the medical literature often leaves something to be desired. Here we will briefly give some tips that can be generally applied. In subsequent chapters we will consider specialised analyses.

For further information Lang and Secic[4] is recommended and they describe a variety of methods for reporting statistics in the medical literature. Checklists for reading and reporting statistical analyses are given in Altman *et al.*[3] For clinical trials the reader is referred to the CONSORT statement.[5]

- Always describe how the subjects were recruited and how many were entered into the study and how many dropped out. For clinical trials one should say how many were screened for entry, and describe the drop-outs by treatment group.

- Describe the model used and assumptions underlying the model and how these were verified.

- Always give an estimate of the main effect, with a measure of precision, such as a 95% confidence interval as well as the P value. It is important to give the right estimate. Thus in a clinical trial, whilst it is of interest to have the mean of the outcome, by treatment group, the main measure of the effect is the difference in means and a confidence interval *for the difference*. This can often not be derived from the confidence intervals of the means for each treatment.

- Describe how the P values were obtained (Wald, likelihood ratio, or score) or the actual tests.

- It is sometimes useful to *describe* the data using binary data (e.g. percentage of people with hypertension), but *analyse* the continuous measurement (e.g. blood pressure).

- Describe which computer package was used. This will often explain why a particular test was used. Results from "home grown" programs may need further verification.

1.11 Reading statistics in the literature

- From what population are the data drawn? Are the results generalisable? Was much of the data missing? Did many people refuse to cooperate?

- Is the analysis confirmatory or exploratory? Is it research or audit?

- Have the correct statistical models been used?

- Do not be satisfied with statements such as "a significant effect was found". Ask what is the size of the effect and will it make a difference to patients (often described as a "clinically significant effect")?

- Are the results critically dependent on the assumptions about the models? Often the results are quite "robust" to the actual model, but this needs to be considered.

Multiple choice questions

1. *Types of data*
A survey of patients with breast cancer was conducted.
Describe the following data as categorical, binary, ordinal, continuous quantitative, and discrete quantitative (count data).

(i) Hospital where patients were treated.
(ii) Age of patient (in years).
(iii) Type of operation.
(iv) Grade of breast cancer.
(v) Heart rate after intense exercise.
(vi) Height.
(vii) Employed/unemployed status.
(viii) Number of visits to a general practitioner per patient per year.

2. *Casual/confounder/outcome variables*
Answer true or false.
In the diet trial described earlier in the chapter:

(i) The outcome variable is weight after treatment.
(ii) Type of diet is a confounding variable.

(iii) Smoking habit is a potential confounding variable.
(iv) Baseline weight could be an input variable.
(v) Diet is a discrete quantitative variable.

3. *Basic statistics*
A trial of cognitive behavioural therapy (CBT) compared to
drug treatment produced the following result: mean depression
score after 6 months, CBT 5.0, drug treatment 6.1, difference
1.1, $P=0.45$, 95% CI –5.0 to 6.2.

(i) CBT is equivalent to drug treatment.
(ii) A possible test to get the P value is the t test.
(iii) The trial is non-significant.
(iv) There is a 45% chance that CBT is better than drug
treatment.
(v) With another trial of the same size under the same
circumstances there is a 95% chance of a mean difference
between −5.0 and 6.2 units.

References

1 Swinscow TDV. *Statistics at Square One, 9th edn.* (revised by MJ
Campbell). London: BMJ Books, 1996.
2 Chatfield C. *Problem Solving. A statistician's guide.* London:
Chapman and Hall, 1995.
3 Altman DG, Machin D, Bryant TN, Gardner MJ eds. *Statistics
with Confidence, 2nd edn.* London: BMJ Books, 2000.
4 Lang TA, Secic M. *How to Report Statistics in Medicine: annotated
guidelines for authors, editors and reviewers.* Philadelphia, PA:
American College of Physicians, 1997.
5 Begg CC, Cho M, Eastwood S, Horton R, Moher D, Olkin I *et
al.* Improving the quality of reporting on randomised controlled
trials: the CONSORT statement. *JAMA*; **276**:1996; 637–9.

2 Multiple linear regression

Summary

When we wish to model an outcome continuous variable, then an appropriate analysis is often *multiple linear regression*. Simple linear regression was covered in Swinscow.[1] For simple linear regression we had one continuous input variable. In multiple regression we generalise the method to more than one input variable and we will allow them to be continuous or categorical. We will discuss the use of *dummy* or *indicator variables* to model categories and investigate the sensitivity of models to individual data points using concepts such as *leverage* and *influence*. Multiple regression is a generalisation of the *analysis of variance* and *analysis of covariance*. The modelling techniques used here will be useful in subsequent chapters.

2.1 The model

In multiple regression the basic model is the following.

$$y_i = \beta_0 + \beta_1 X_{i1} + \beta_2 X_{i2} + \ldots + \beta_k X_{ik} + \varepsilon_i . \qquad (2.1)$$

We assume that the error term ε_i is Normally distributed, with mean zero and standard deviation σ.

In terms of the model structure described in Chapter 1, the link is a linear one and the error term is Normal.

Here y_i is the output for unit or subject i and there are k input variables $X_{i1}, X_{i2},\ldots,X_{ik}$. Often y_i is termed the *dependent* variable and the input variables $X_{i1}, X_{i2},\ldots,X_{ik}$ are termed the *independent variables*. The latter can be continuous or nominal. However the term "independent" is a misnomer since the Xs need not be independent of each other. Sometimes they are called the *explanatory* or *predictor* variables. Each of the input variables is associated with a *regression coefficient* β_1, β_2,...β_k. There is also an additive constant term β_0. These are the *model parameters*.

We can write the first section on the right hand side of equation (2.1) as

$$LP_i = \beta_0 + \beta_1 X_{i1} + \beta_2 X_{i2} + ... + \beta_k X_{ik}$$

where LP_i is known as the *linear predictor* and is the value of y_i predicted by the input variables. The difference $y_i - LP_i = \varepsilon_i$ is the *error* term.

The models are fitted by choosing estimates b_0, b_1,...b_k which minimise the sum of squares of the predicted error. These estimates are termed *ordinary least squares* estimates. Using these estimates we can calculate the fitted values y_i^{fit}, and the observed residuals $e_i = y_i - y_i^{fit}$ as discussed in Chapter 1. Here it is clear that the residuals estimate the error term. Further details are given in Draper and Smith.[2]

2.2 Uses of multiple regression

1. To adjust the effects of an input variable on a continuous output variable for the effects of confounders. For example, to investigate the effect of diet on weight allowing for smoking habits. Here the dependent variable is the outcome from a clinical trial. The independent variables could be the two treatment groups (as a 0/1 binary variable), smoking (as a continuous variable in numbers of packs per week) and baseline weight. The multiple regression allows one to compare the outcome between groups, allowing for differences in baseline and smoking habit.

2. For predicting a value of an outcome, for given inputs. For example, an investigator might wish to predict the FEV_1 of a subject given age and height, so as to be able to calculate the observed FEV_1 as a percentage of predicted and to decide if the observed FEV_1 is below, say, 80% of the predicted one.

3. To analyse the simultaneous effects of a number of categorical variables on an output variable. An alternative technique is the *analysis of variance* but the same results can be achieved using multiple regression.

2.3 Two independent variables

We will start off by considering two independent variables which can be either continuous or binary. There are three possibilities: both variables continuous, both binary (0/1) or one continuous and one binary. We will anchor the examples in some real data.

Example

Consider the data given on the pulmonary anatomical deadspace and height in 15 children given in Swinscow.[1] Suppose that of the 15 children, 8 had asthma and 4 bronchitis. The data are given in Table 2.1

Table 2.1 Lung function data on 15 children.

Child number	Deadspace (ml)	Height (cm)	Asthma (0=No,) 1=Yes)	Age (Years)	Bronchitis (0=No, 1=Yes)
1	44	110	1	5	0
2	31	116	0	5	1
3	43	124	1	6	0
4	45	129	1	7	0
5	56	131	1	7	0
6	79	138	0	6	0
7	57	142	1	6	0
8	56	150	1	8	0
9	58	153	1	8	0
10	92	155	0	9	1
11	78	156	0	7	1
12	64	159	1	8	0
13	88	164	0	10	1
14	112	168	0	11	0
15	101	174	0	14	0

2.3.1 One continuous and one binary independent variable

In Swinscow,[1] the problem posed was whether there is a relationship between deadspace and height. Here we might ask, is there a different relationship between deadspace and height for asthmatics than for non-asthmatics?

Here we have two independent variables, height and asthma status. There are a number of possible models:

1. *The slope and the intercept are the same for the two groups even though the means are different.*

The model is

$$\text{Deadspace} = \beta_0 + \beta_{\text{Height}} \times \text{Height} \qquad (2.2)$$

This is illustrated in Figure 2.1. This is the simple linear regression model described in Swinscow.[1]

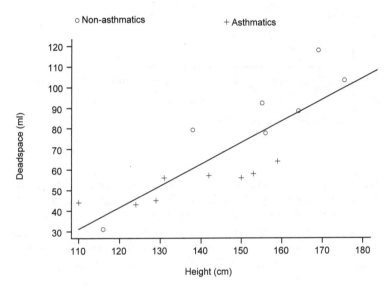

Figure 2.1 Deadspace versus height ignoring asthma status.

2. *The slopes are the same, but the intercepts are different.*

The model is

$$\text{Deadspace} = \beta_0 + \beta_{\text{Height}} \times \text{Height} + \beta_{\text{Asthma}} \times \text{Asthma} \qquad (2.3)$$

This is illustrated in Figure 2.2. It can be seen from model (2.3) that the interpretation of the coefficient β_{Asthma} is the difference in the intercepts of the two parallel lines which have slope β_{Height}. It is the difference in deadspace between asthmatics and non-

15

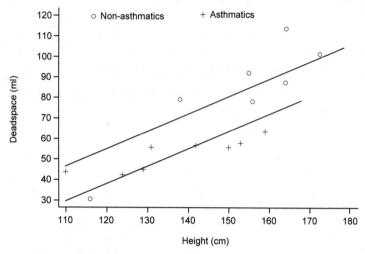

Figure 2.2 Parallel slopes for asthmatics and non-asthmatics.

asthmatics for any value of height, or to put it another way, it is the difference *allowing for* height. Thus if we thought that the only reason that asthmatics and non-asthmatics in our sample differed in the deadspace was because of a difference in height, this is the sort of model we would fit. This type of model is termed an *analysis of covariance*. It is very common in the medical literature. An important assumption is that the slope is the same for the two groups.

We shall see later that, although they have the same symbol, we will get different estimates of β_{Height} when we fit (2.2) and (2.3).

3. *The slopes and the intercepts are different in each group.*

To model this we form a third variable $x_3 =$ Height$\times$Asthma. Thus x_3 is the same as height when the subject is asthmatic and is zero otherwise. The variable x_3 measures the *interaction* between asthma status and height. It measures by how much the slope between deadspace and height is affected by being an asthmatic.

The model is

Deadspace=
$\beta_0 + \beta_{Height} \times Height + \beta_{Asthma} \times Asthma + \beta_3 \times Height \times Asthma$ (2.4)

This is illustrated in Figure 2.3. In this graph we have separate slopes for non-asthmatics and asthmatics.

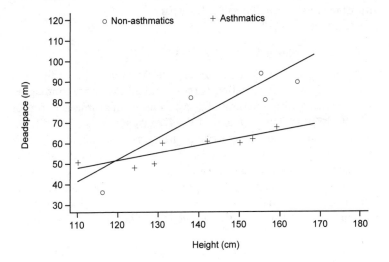

Figure 2.3 Separate lines for asthmatics and non-asthmatics.

The two lines are:
Non-asthmatics

Group=0: Deadspace=$\beta_0 + \beta_{Height} \times Height$

Asthmatics

Group=1: Deadspace=$(\beta_0 + \beta_{Asthma}) + (\beta_{Height} + \beta_3) \times Height$

In this model the interpretation of β_{Height} has changed from model (2.3). It is now the slope of the expected line for non-

17

asthmatics. The slope of the line for asthmatics is $\beta_{Height}+\beta_3$. We then get the difference in slopes between asthmatics and non-asthmatics is given by β_3.

2.3.2 Two continuous independent variables

As an example of a situation where both independent variables are continuous, consider the data given in Table 2.1, but suppose we were interested in whether height and age together were important in the prediction of deadspace.

The equation is

$$Deadspace = \beta_0 + \beta_1 \times Height + \beta_2 \times Age.$$

The interpretation of this model is trickier than the earlier one and the graphical visualisation is more difficult. We have to imagine that we have a whole variety of subjects all of the same age, but of different heights. Then we expect the Deadspace to go up by β_1 ml for each cm in height, irrespective of the ages of the subjects. We also have to imagine a group of subjects, all of the same height, but different ages. Then we expect the Deadspace to go up by β_2 ml for each year of age, irrespective of the heights of the subjects. The nice feature of the model is that we can estimate these coefficients reasonably even if none of the subjects has exactly the same age, or height.

This model is commonly used in prediction as described in section 2.2.

2.3.3 Categorical independent variables

In Table 2.1, the way that asthmatic status was coded is known as a *dummy* or *indicator variable*. There are two levels, asthmatic and non-asthmatic, and just one dummy variable, the coefficient of which measures the difference in the y variable between asthmatics and normals. For inference it does not matter if we code 1 for asthmatics and 0 for normals or vice versa. The only effect is to change the sign of the coefficient; the P value will remain the same. However the table describes three categories: asthmatic, bronchitic and neither (taken as normal!), and these categories are mutually exclusive (i.e. there are no children with both asthma and bronchitis). Table 2.2 gives possible dummy variables for a group of three subjects.

Table 2.2 *One method of coding a three-category variable.*

Status	x_1	x_2	x_3
Asthmatic	1	0	0
Bronchitic	0	1	0
Normal	0	0	1

We now have three possible contrasts asthmatics vs bronchitics, asthmatics vs normals and bronchitics vs normals, but they are not all independent. Knowing two of the contrasts we can deduce the third (if you are not asthmatic or bronchitic you *must* be normal!). Thus we need to choose two of the three contrasts to include in the regression and thus two dummy variables to include in a regression. If we included all three variables, most regression programs would inform us politely that x_1, x_2 and x_3 were *aliased* (i.e. mutually dependent) and omit one of the variables from the equation. The dummy variable that is omitted from the regression is the one that the coefficients for the other variables are contrasted with, and is known as the *baseline* variable. Thus if x_3 is omitted in the regression which includes x_1 and x_2 in Table 2.2, then the coefficient attached to x_1 is the difference between deadspace for asthmatics and normals. Another way of looking at it is that the coefficient associated with the baseline is constrained to be zero.

2.4 Interpreting a computer output

We now describe how to interpret a computer output for linear regression. Most statistical packages produce an output similar to this one. The models are fitted using the *principle of least squares*, which is explained in Appendix 2, and is equivalent to maximum likelihood when the error distribution is Normal.

2.4.1 One continuous and one binary independent variable

We must first create a new variable Asthma=1 for asthmatics and Asthma=0 for non-asthmatics and create a new variable AsthmaHt=Asthma×Height for the interaction of asthma and height. Some packages can do both of these automatically if one declares asthma as a "factor" or as "categorical", and fits a term such as Asthma*Height in the model.

The results of fitting these variables using a computer program are given in Table 2.3

Table 2.3 Output from computer program fitting height and asthma status and their interaction to deadspace from Table 2.1.

Source	SS	df	MS	
				Number of obs = 15
				F(3, 11) = 37.08
Model	7124.3865	3	2374.7955	Prob > F = 0.0000
Residual	704.546834	11	64.0497122	R-squared = 0.9100
				Adj R-squared = 0.8855
Total	7828.93333	14	559.209524	Root MSE = 8.0031

Deadspace	Coef.	Std. Err.	t	P>|t|	[95% Conf. Interval]	
Height	1.192565	.1635673	7.291	0.000	.8325555	1.552574
Asthma	95.47263	35.61056	2.681	0.021	17.09433	173.8509
AsthmaHt	−.7782494	.2447751	−3.179	0.009	−1.316996	−.239503
_cons	−99.46241	25.20795	−3.946	0.002	−154.9447	−43.98009

We fit three independent variables Height, Asthma and AsthmaHt on Deadspace. This is equivalent to model (2.4), and is shown in Figure 2.3. The computer program gives two sections of output. The first part refers to fit of the overall model. The $F(3,11) = 37.08$ is what is known as an F statistic (after the statistician Fisher), which depends on two numbers which are known as the *degrees of freedom*. The first, k, is the number of parameters in the model (excluding the constant term β_0) which in this case is 3 and the second is $n-k-1$ where n is the number of subjects and in this case is $15-3-1=11$. The Prob > F is the probability that the variability associated with the model could have occurred by chance, on the assumption that the true model has only a constant term and no explanatory variables, in other words the overall significance of the model. This is given as 0.0000, which we interpret as $P < 0.0001$. It means that fitting all three variables *simultaneously* gives a highly significant fit. It does *not* tell us about individual variables. An important statistic is the value R^2, which is the proportion of variance of the original data explained by the model and in this model is 0.91. For models with only one independent variable it is simply the square of the correlation coefficient described in Swinscow.[1] However, one can always obtain an arbitrarily good fit by fitting as many parameters as there are observations. To allow for this, we calculate the R^2 *adjusted for degrees of freedom*, which is $R^2_a = 1 - (1 - R^2)(n-1)/(n-k)$ and in this case is given by 0.89. The root MSE means the "residual mean square error" and has the value 8.0031. It is an estimate of σ in equation (2.1) and can be deduced as the square root of the residual MS (mean square) in left-hand table. Thus $\sqrt{64.0497} = 8.0031$.

The second part of the output examines the individual coefficients in the model. We see that the interaction term between height and asthma status is significant ($P = 0.009$). The *difference* in the slopes is -0.778 units (95% CI -1.317 to -0.240). There are no terms to drop from the model. Note, even if one of the main terms, asthma or height was not significant, we would *not* drop it from the model if the interaction was significant, since the interaction cannot be interpreted in the absence of the main effects, which in this case are asthma and height.

The two lines of best fit are:

Non-asthmatics:

$$\text{Deadspace} = -99.46 + 1.193 \times \text{Height}$$

Asthmatics:

$$\text{Deadspace} = (-99.46 + 95.47) + (1.193 - 0.778) \times \text{Height}$$
$$= -3.99 + 0.425 \times \text{Height}$$

Thus the deadspace in asthmatics appears to grow more slowly with height than that of non-asthmatics.

Quite clearly, the intercepts for these equations are meaningless. They are the projected values of deadspace assuming the subject had no height and are completely uninterpretable.

2.4.2 Two independent variables: both continuous

Here we were interested in whether height or age were both important in the prediction of deadspace. The analysis is given in Table 2.4.

The equation is

$$\text{Deadspace} = -59.05 + 0.707 \times \text{Height} + 3.045 \times \text{Age}$$

The interpretation of this model is described in section 2.3.2. Note a peculiar feature of this output. Although the overall model is significant ($P = 0.0003$) neither of the coefficients associated with height and age are significant (P = 0.063 and 0.291 respectively!). This occurs because age and height are strongly correlated and highlights the importance of looking at the overall fit of a model. Dropping either will leave the other as a significant predictor in the model. Note that if we drop age, the adjusted R^2 is not greatly affected ($R^2 = 0.6944$ for height alone compared to 0.6995 for age and height) suggesting that height is a better predictor.

Table 2.4 Output from computer program fitting age and height to deadspace from Table 2.1.

Source	SS	df	MS					
				Number of obs	=	15		
				F(2, 12)	=	17.29		
Model	5812.17397	2	2906.08698	Prob > F	=	0.0003		
Residual	2016.75936	12	168.06328	R-squared	=	0.7424		
				Adj R-squared	=	0.6995		
Total	7828.93333	14	559.209524	Root MSE	=	12.964		

Deadspace	Coef.	Std. Err.	t	P>|t|	[95% Conf. Interval]	
Height	.7070318	.3455362	2.046	0.063	−.0458268	1.45989
Age	3.044691	2.758517	1.104	0.291	−2.965602	9.054984
_cons	−59.05205	33.63162	−1.756	0.105	−132.329	14.22495

Bootstrap statistics

Variable	Reps	Observed	Bias	Std. Err.	[95% Conf. Interval]		
Height	1000	.7070318	−.0080937	.3313434	.056823	1.357241	(N)
					.0793041	1.312535	(P)
					.0845788	1.31849	(BC)
Age	1000	3.044691	.3040586	3.399811	−3.6269	9.716281	(N)
					−2.586633	10.66853	(P)
					−2.986388	10.29889	(BC)

N = normal, P = percentile, BC = bias-corrected

2.4.3 Use of a bootstrap estimate

In the lower half of Table 2.4 we illustrate the use of a computer-intensive method, known as a *bootstrap,* to provide a more robust estimate of the standard error of the regression coefficients. The basis for the bootstrap is described in Appendix 3.

This method is less dependent on distributional assumptions

than the usual methods described in this book and involves sampling the data a large number of times and recalculating the regression equation on each occasion. It would be used, for example, if a plot of the residuals indicated a marked asymmetry in their distribution. The computer program produces three alternative estimators, a Normal estimate – a percentile estimate (PC) and a bias-corrected estimate (BC). We recommend the last. It can be seen that a bootstrap estimate for the standard error of the height estimate is slightly smaller than the conventional estimate, so that the confidence intervals no longer include 0. The bootstrap standard error for age is larger. This would confirm our earlier conclusion that height is the stronger predictor here.

2.4.4 Categorical independent variables

It will help the interpretation to know that the mean values (ml) for deadspace for the three groups are normals 97.33, asthmatics 52.88 and bronchitics 72.25. The analysis is given in Table 2.5. Here the two independent variables are x_1 and x_2 in Table 2.3. As

Table 2.5 Output from computer program fitting two categorical variables to deadspace from Table 2.2.

Asthma and bronchitis as independent variables

Number of obs = 15, F(2,12) = 7.97,Prob > F = 0.0063
R-squared = 0.5705 Adj R-squared = 0.4990

y	Coef.	Std. Err.	t	P>|t|	[95% Conf. Interval]	
Asthma	−44.45833	11.33229	−3.923	0.002	−69.14928	−19.76739
Bronch	−25.08333	12.78455	−1.962	0.073	−52.93848	2.771809
_cons	97.33333	9.664212	10.072	0.000	76.27683	118.3898

Asthma and Normal as independent variables

Number of obs =15, F(2, 12) = 7.97, Prob > F = 0.0063
R-squared = 0.5705, Adj R-squared = 0.4990

y	Coef.	Std. Err.	t	P>|t|	[95% Conf. Interval]	
Asthma	−19.375	10.25044	−1.890	0.083	−41.7088	2.9588
Normal	25.08333	12.78455	1.962	0.073	−2.771809	52.93848
_cons	72.25	8.369453	8.633	0.000	54.01453	90.48547

we noted before an important point to check is that in general one should see that the overall model is significant, before looking at the individual contrasts. Here we have Prob > F = 0.0063, which means that the overall model is highly significant. If we look at the individual contrasts we see that the coefficient associated with asthma, −44.46, is the difference in means between normals and asthmatics. This has a standard error of 11.33 and so is highly significant. The coefficient associated with bronchitics, −25.08, is the contrast between bronchitics and normals and is not significant, implying that the mean deadspace is not significantly different in bronchitics and normals.

If we wished to contrast asthmatics and bronchitics, we need to make one of them the baseline. Thus we use x_1 and x_3 as the independent variables to make bronchitics the baseline and the output is shown in Table 2.5. As would be expected the Prob > F and the R^2 value are the same as the earlier model because these refer to the overall model which differs from the earlier one only in the formulation of the parameters. However, now the coefficients refer to the contrast with bronchitics, and we can see that the difference between asthmatics and bronchitics has a difference −19.38 with standard error 10.25, which is not significant.

Thus the only significant difference is between asthmatics and normals.

This method of analysis is also known as *one-way analysis of variance*. It is a generalisation of the *t* test referred to in Swinscow.[1] One could ask what is the difference between this and simply carrying out two *t* tests, asthmatics vs normals and bronchitics vs normals. In fact the analysis of variance accomplishes two extra refinements. Firstly, the overall P value controls for the problem of multiple testing referred to in Swinscow.[1] By doing a number of tests against the baseline we are increasing the chances of a Type I error. The overall P value in the F test allows for this and since it is significant, we know that some of the contrasts must be significant. The second improvement is that in order to calculate a *t* test we must find the pooled standard error. In the *t* test this is done from two groups, whereas in the analysis of variance it is calculated from all three, which is based on more subjects and so is more precise.

2.5 Multiple regression in action

2.5.1 Analysis of covariance

We mentioned that model (2.3) is very commonly seen in the literature. To see its application in a clinical trial consider the results of Llewellyn-Jones et al.,[3] part of which are given in Table 2.6. This study was a randomised controlled trial of the effectiveness of a shared care intervention for depression in 220 subjects over the age of 65. Depression was measured using the Geriatric Depression Scale, taken at baseline and after 9.5 months of blinded follow up. The figure that helps the interpretation is Figure 2.2. Here y is the depression scale after 9.5 months of treatment (continuous), x_1 is the value of the same scale at baseline and x_2 is the group variable, taking the value 1 for intervention and 0 for control.

The *standardised regression coefficient* is not universally defined, but in this case is obtained when the x variable is replaced by x divided by its standard deviation. Thus the interpretation of the standardised regression coefficient is the amount the y changes for one standard deviation increase in x. One can see that the baseline values are highly correlated with the follow-up values of the score. The intervention resulted on average, in patients with a score 1.87 units (95% CI 0.76 to 2.97) lower than those in the control group, throughout the range of the baseline values.

Table 2.6 Factors affecting Geriatric Depression Scale score at follow up.

Variable	Regression coefficient (95% CI)	Standardised regression coefficient	P value
Baseline score	0.73 (0.56 to 0.91)	0.56	<0.0001
Treatment group	−1.87 (-2.97 to -0.76)	−0.22	0.0011

This analysis assumes that the treatment effect is the same for all subjects and is not related to values of their baseline scores. This possibility could be checked by the methods discussed earlier. When two groups are balanced with respect to the baseline value, one might assume that including the baseline value in the analysis will not affect the comparison of treatment groups. However, it is often worthwhile including because it can improve the precision of the estimate of the treatment effect, i.e. the standard errors of the treatment effects may be smaller when the baseline covariate is included.

2.5.2 Two continuous independent variables

Sorensen et al.[4] describe a cohort study of 4300 men, aged between 18 and 26, who had their body mass index (BMI) measured. The investigators wished to relate adult BMI to the men's birthweight and body length at birth. Potential confounding factors included gestational age, birth order, mother's marital status, age and occupation. In a multiple linear regression they found an association between birthweight (coded in units of 250 g) and BMI (allowing for confounders), regression coefficient 0.82, SE 0.17, but not between birth length (cm) and BMI, regression coefficient 1.51, SE 3.87. Thus for every increase in birthweight of 250 g, the BMI increases on average by 0.82 kg/m^2. The authors suggest that *in utero* factors that affect birthweight continue to have an effect even into adulthood, even allowing for factors such as gestational age.

2.6 Assumptions underlying the models

There are a number of assumptions implicit in the choice of the model. The most fundamental assumption is that the model is *linear*. This means that each increase by one unit of an x variable is associated with a fixed increase in the y variable, irrespective of the starting value of the x variable.

There are a number of ways of checking this when x is continuous:

- For single continuous independent variables the simplest check is a visual one from a scatter plot of y versus x.

- Try transformations of the x variables ($\log(x)$, x^2 and $1/x$ are the commonest). There is not a simple significance test for one transformation against another, but a good guide would be if the R^2 value gets larger.

- Include a quadratic term (x^2) as well as the linear term (x) in the model. This model is the one where we fit two continuous variables x and x^2. A significant coefficient for x^2 indicates a lack of linearity.

- Divide x into a number of groups such as by quintiles. Fit separate dummy variables for the four largest quintile groups and examine the coefficients. For a linear relationship, the coefficients themselves will increase linearly.

Another fundamental assumption is that the error terms are independent of each other. An example of where this is unlikely is when the data form a time series. A simple check for sequential data for independent errors is whether the residuals are correlated, and a test known as the *Durbin-Watson test* is available in many packages. Further details are given in Chapter 6, on time-series analysis. A further example of lack of independence is where the main unit of measurement is the individual, but that several observations are made on each individual, and these are treated as if they came from different individuals. This is the problem of *repeated measures*. A similar type of problem occurs when groups of patients are randomised, rather than individual patients. These are discussed in Chapter 5, on repeated measures.

The model also assumes that the error terms are independent of the x variables and variance of the error term is constant (the latter goes under the more complicated term of *heteroscedascity*). A common alternative is when the error increases as one of the x variables increases, so one way of checking this assumption would be to plot the residuals, e_i against each of the independent variables and also against the fitted values. If the model were correct one would expect to see the scatter of residuals evenly spread about the horizontal axis and not showing any pattern. A common departure from this is when the residuals fan out, i.e. the scatter gets larger as the x variable gets larger. This is often also associated with non-linearity as well, and so attempts at transforming the x variable may resolve the issue.

The final assumption is that the error term is Normally distributed. One could check this by plotting a histogram of the residuals, although the method of fitting will mean that the observed residuals e_i are likely to be closer to a Normal distribution than the true ones ε_i. The assumption of Normality is important mainly so that we can use normal theory to estimate confidence intervals around the coefficients, but luckily with reasonably large sample sizes, the estimation method is robust to departures from normality. Thus moderate departures from Normality are allowable. One could also use bootstrap methods described in Appendix 3.

It is important to remember that the main purpose of the analysis is to assess a relationship, *not* test assumptions, so often we can come to a useful conclusion *even when the assumptions are not perfectly satisfied.*

2.7 Model sensitivity

Model sensitivity refers to how estimates are affected by subgroups of the data. Suppose we had fitted a simple regression (model 2.2), and we were told that the estimates b_0 and b_1 altered dramatically if you deleted a subset of the data, or even a single individual. This is important, because we like to think that the model applies generally, and we don't wish to find that we should have different models for different subgroups of patients.

2.7.1 Residuals, leverage and influence

There are three main issues in identifying model sensitivity to individual observations: *residuals, leverage* and *influence.* The residuals are the difference between the observed and fitted data $e_i = y_i^{obs} - y_i^{fit}$. A point with a large residual is called an *outlier.* In general we are interested in outliers because they may influence the estimates, but it is possible to have a large outlier which is not influential.

Another way that a point can be an outlier is if the values of x_i are a long way from the mass of each x. For a single variable, this means if x_i is a long way from $\bar{x}$. Imagine a scatter plot of y against x, with a mass of points in the bottom left hand corner and a single point in the top right. It is possible that this individual has unique characteristics which relate to both the x and y variables. A regression line fitted to the data will go close, or even through the isolated point. This isolated point will not have a large residual, yet if this point is deleted the regression coefficient might change dramatically. Such a point is said to have *high leverage* and this can be measured by a number, often denoted h_i where large values of h_i indicate a high leverage.

An influential point is one that has a large effect on an estimate.

Effectively one fits the model with and without that point and finds the effect of the regression coefficient. One might look for points that have a large effect on b_0, or on b_1 or on other estimates such as $SE(b_1)$. The usual output is the difference in the regression coefficient for a particular variable when the point is included or excluded, scaled by the estimated standard error of the coefficient. The problem is that different parameters may have different influential points. Most computer packages now produce residuals, leverages, and influential points as a matter of routine. It is the task for an analyst to examine these and identify important cases. However, just because a case is influential or has a large residual it does not follow that it should be deleted, although the data should be examined carefully for possible measurement or transcription errors. A proper analysis of such data would report such sensitivities to individual points.

2.7.2 Computer analysis: model checking and sensitivity

We will illustrate model checking and sensitivity using the deadspace, age and height data in Table 2.1.

Figure 2.1 gives us reassurance that the relationship between deadspace and height is plausibly linear. We could plot a similar graph for deadspace and age. The standard diagnostic plot is a plot of the residuals against the fitted values, and for the model fitted in Table 2.3 it is shown in Figure 2.4. There is no apparent pattern, which gives us reassurance about the error term being relatively constant and further reassurance about the linearity of the model.

The diagnostic statistics are shown in Table 2.7 where the *influence* statistics are *inf_age* associated with age and *inf_ht* associated with height. As one might expect the children with the highest leverages are the youngest (who is also the shortest) and the oldest (who is also the tallest). Notice that the largest residuals are associated with small leverages. This is because points with large leverage will tend to force the line close to them.

The child with the most influence on the age coefficient is also the oldest, and removal of that child would change the standardised regression coefficient by 0.79 units. The child with the most influence on height is the shortest child. However, neither child should be removed without strong reason. (A strong reason may be if it was discovered the child had some relevant disease, such as cystic fibrosis.)

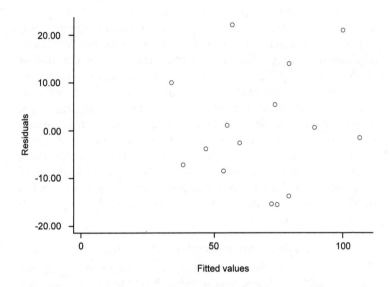

Figure 2.4 Graph of residuals against fitted values for regression model in Table 2.4 with age and height as the independent variables

Table 2.7 Diagnostics from model fitted in Table 2.4 (output from computer program)

	Height	Age	resids	leverage	inf_age	inf_ht
1.	110	5	10.06	0.33	0.22	−0.48
2.	116	5	−7.19	0.23	−0.04	0.18
3.	124	6	−3.89	0.15	−0.03	0.08
4.	129	7	−8.47	0.15	−0.14	0.20
5.	131	7	1.12	0.12	0.01	−0.02
6.	138	6	22.21	0.13	−0.52	0.34
7.	142	6	−2.61	0.17	0.08	−0.06
8.	150	8	−15.36	0.08	0.11	−0.14
9.	153	8	−15.48	0.10	0.20	−0.26
10.	155	9	14.06	0.09	0.02	0.07
11.	156	7	5.44	0.28	−0.24	0.25
12.	159	8	−13.72	0.19	0.38	−0.46
13.	164	10	0.65	0.14	0.00	0.01
14.	168	11	18.78	0.19	0.29	0.08
15.	174	14	−5.60	0.65	−0.79	0.42

2.8 Stepwise regression

When one has a large number of independent variables, a natural question to ask is, what is the best combination of these variables to predict the y variable? To answer this one may use *stepwise regression* which is available in a number of packages. *Step-down* or *backwards regression* starts by fitting all available variables and then discarding sequentially those that are not significant. *Step-up* or *forwards regression* starts by fitting an overall mean, and then selecting variables to add to the model according to their significance. *Stepwise regression* is a mixture of the two, where one can specify a P value for a variable to be entered into the model, and then a P value for a variable to be discarded. Usually one chooses a larger P value for entry (say 0.1) than for exclusion (say 0.05), since variables can jointly be predictive, when separately they are not. This also favours step-down regression. As an example consider an outcome variable being the amount a person limps. Neither the length of the left or right legs are predictive, but the difference in lengths is highly predictive. Stepwise regression is best used in the *exploratory phase* of an analysis (see Chapter 1), to identify a few predictors in a mass of data, the association of which can be verified by further data collection.

There are a few problems with stepwise regression:

- The P values are invalid since they do not take account of the vast number of tests that have been carried out; different methods such as step-up and step-down are likely to produce different models and experience shows that the same model rarely emerges when a second data set is analysed. One way of trying to counter this is to split a large data set into two, and run the stepwise procedure on both separately. Choose the variables that are common to both data sets, and fit these to the combined data sets as the final model.

- Many large data sets contain missing values. With stepwise regression, usually only the subjects who have no missing values on *any* of the variables under consideration are chosen. The final model may contain only a few variables, but if one refits the model, the parameters change because now the model is being fitted to those subjects who have no missing values on only the few chosen variables, which may be a considerably larger data set than the original.

- If a categorical variable is coded as a number of dummies, some of these may be lost in the fitting process, and this changes the interpretation of the others. Thus if we fitted x_1 and x_2 from Table 2.2, and then we lost x_2, the interpretation of x_1 is of a contrast between asthmatics with bronchitics and normals *combined*.

Thus stepwise regression is useful in the exploratory phase of an analysis, but not the *confirmatory* phase.

2.9 Reporting the results of a multiple regression

- As a minimum, report the regression coefficients and standard errors or confidence intervals for the main independent variables, together with the adjusted R^2 for the whole model.

- If a bootstrap estimate of the confidence interval is being used, state the method used (e.g. bias corrected) and the number of replications.

- If there is one main dependent variable, show a scatter plot of each independent variable versus the dependent variable with the best fit line.

- Report how the assumptions underlying the model were tested and verified. In particular is linearity plausible?

- Report any sensitivity analysis carried out.

- Report *all* the variables included in the model. For a stepwise regression, report *all* the variables that could have entered the model.

- Note that if an interaction term is included in a model, the main effects *must* be included.

2.10 Reading the results of a multiple regression

In addition to the points in section 1.11.

- Note the value of R^2. With a large study, the coefficients in the model can be highly significant, but only explain a low proportion of the variability of the outcome variable. Thus they may be no use for prediction.

- Are the models plausibly linear? Are there any boundaries, which may cause the slope to flatten?

- Were outliers and influential points identified and how were they treated?

- An analysis of covariance *assumes* that the slopes are the same in each group. Is this plausible and has it been tested?

Frequently asked questions

1. Does it matter how a dummy variable is coded?
If you have only one binary variable, then coding the dummy variable 0 and 1 is the most convenient. Coding it 1 and 2 is commonly the method in questionnaires. It will make no difference to the coefficient estimate or P value. However it will change the value of the intercept, because now the value in the group assigned 1 will be $a+b$ and the value in the group assigned 2 will be $a+2b$. Thus in Figure 2.2 when "Asthma" is coded 0 or 1 the regression coefficient for Asthma is -16.8 and the intercept is -46.3. If we had coded the variable 1 or 2 we would find the regression coefficient for Asthma is still -16.8 but the intercept would be $(-46.3-16.8) = -63.1$. Coding the dummy variable to -1 and $+1$ (as is done for example in the package SAS) does not change the P value but the coefficient is halved.

If you have a categorical variable with, say, three groups, then this will be coded with two dummy variables. As shown earlier, the overall F statistic will be unchanged no matter which two groups are chosen to be represented by dummies, but the coefficient of group 2, say, will be dependent on whether group 1 or group 3 is the omitted variable.

2. How do I treat an ordinal independent variable?
Most packages assume that the predictor variable, X, in a regression model is either continuous or binary. Thus one has a number of options.

(i) Treat the predictor as if it were continuous. This incorporates into the model the fact that the categories are ordered, but also assumes that equal changes in X mean equal changes in y.

(ii) Treat the predictor as if it were categorical, by fitting dummy variables to all but one of the categories. This loses the fact that the predictor is ordinal, but makes no assumption about linearity.

(iii) Dichotomise the X variable, by recoding it as binary, say 1 if y is in a particular category or above, and zero otherwise. The cut point should be chosen on external grounds and not because it gives the best fit to the data.

Which of these options you choose depends on a number of factors. With a large amount of data, the loss of information by ignoring the ordinality in option (ii) is not critical and especially if the X variable is a confounder and not of prime interest. For example, if X is age grouped in 10-year intervals, it might be better to fit dummy variables, than assume a linear relation with the y variable.

3. Do the assumptions underlying multiple regression matter?
Often the assumptions underlying multiple regression are not checked, partly because the investigator is confident that they hold true and partly because mild departures are unlikely to invalidate an analysis. However, lack of independence may be obvious on empirical grounds (the data form repeated measures or a time series) and so the analysis should accommodate this from the outset. Linearity is important for inference and so may be checked by fitting transformations of the independent variables. Lack of homogeneity of variance and lack of normality may affect the standard errors and often indicate the need for a transformation of the dependent variable. The most common departure from Normality is when outliers are identified, and these should be carefully checked, particularly those with high leverage.

4. I have a variable that I believe should be a confounder but it is not significant. Should I include it in the analysis?
There are certain variables (such as age or sex) for which one might have strong grounds for believing that they could be confounders, but in any particular analysis may emerge as significant. These should be retained in the analysis because, even if not significantly related to the outcome themselves, they may modify the effect of the prime independent variable.

5. *What happens if I have a dependent variable which is 0 or 1?*
When the dependent variable is 0 or 1 then the coefficients from a linear regression are proportional to what is known as the *linear discriminant function*. This can be useful for discriminating between groups, even if the assumption about Normality of the residuals is violated. However discrimination is normally carried out now using *logistic regression* (Chapter 3).

Multiple choice questions

1. Ross *et al.*[5] regressed mortality in working aged men against median share of income (i.e. the proportion of total income accruing to the less well off 50% of households) in 282 USA metropolitan areas and 53 Canadian metropolitan areas. The median income for the areas was included as an explanatory variable. They found the difference in slopes significant $(P < 0.01)$, $R^2 = 0.51$.

The model is
$$yi = a + b_1 X_{1i} + b_2 X_{2i} + b_3 X_{3i} + b_4 X_{4i}$$

y_i is the mortality per 100 000 for metropolitan area i, $i = 1...335$
X_{1i} takes the value 1 for the USA and 0 for Canada
X_{2i} is median share of income for area i (defined above)
$X_{3i} = X_{i1}.X_{2i}$ (the product of X_{1i} and X_{2i})
X_{4i} is median income for area i

(i)   Mortality is assumed to have a Normal distribution.
(ii) The test to compare slopes is a t test with 330 degrees of freedom.
(iii) The relationship between mortality and median income is assumed to be different for the USA and Canada.
(iv) The relationship between mortality and median share of income is assumed linear.
(v)   The variability of the residuals is assumed the same for the USA and Canada.

2. In a multiple regression equation $y = a + b_1 X_1 + b_2 X_2$,

(i)   The independent variables X_1 and X_2 must be continuous

(ii) The leverage depends on the values of y.
(iii) The slope b_2 is unaffected by values of X_1.
(iv) If X_2 is a categorical variable with three categories, it is modelled by two dummy variables.
(v) If there are 100 points in the data set, then there are 97 degrees of freedom for testing b_1.

References

1 Swinscow TDV. *Statistics at Square One, 9th edn.* (revised by MJ Campbell). London: BMJ Books, 1996.
2 Draper NR, Smith H. *Applied Regression Analysis, 3rd edn.* New York: John Wiley, 1998.
3 Llewellyn-Jones RH, Baikie KA, Smithers H, Cohen J, Snowdon J, Tennant CC. Multifaceted shared care intervention for late life depression in residential care: randomised controlled trial. *BMJ* 1999; **319**: 676–82.
4 Sorensen HT, Sabroe S, Rothman KJ, Gillman M, Fischer P, Sorensen TIA. Relation between weight and length at birth and body mass index in young adulthood: cohort study. *BMJ* 1997; **315:** 1137.
5 Ross NA, Wolfson MC, Dunn JR, Berthelot J-M, Kaplan GA, Lynch JW. Relation between income inequality and mortality in Canada and in the United States: cross-sectional assessment using census data and vital statistics. *BMJ* 2000; **320**: 898-902.

3 Logistic regression

Summary

When we wish to model a binary dependent variable, then an appropriate analysis is often *logistic regression*. In Swinscow[1] we described the chi-squared test for testing the association of two binary variables. Logistic regression is a generalisation of the chi-squared test to examine the association of a binary-dependent variable with one or more independent variables which can be binary, categorical (more than two categories) or continuous. Logistic regression is also useful for analysing *case-control studies*. Matched case-control studies require a particular analysis known as *conditional logistic regression*.

3.1 The model

The dependent variable can be described as an *event* which is either present or absent (sometimes termed "success" and "failure"). Thus an event might be the presence of a disease in a survey or cure from disease in a clinical trial. We wish to examine factors associated with the event. Since we can rarely predict exactly whether an event will happen or not, what we in fact look for are factors associated with the *probability* of an event happening.

There are two situations to consider:

1. Firstly, when all the independent variables are categorical, and so one can form tables in which each cell has individuals with the same values of the independent variables. As a consequence one can calculate the proportion of subjects for whom an event happens. For example, one might wish to examine the presence or absence of a disease by gender (two categories) and social class (five categories). Thus one could

form a table with the 10 social class-by-gender categories and examine the proportion of subjects with disease in each grouping.

2. Secondly, when the data table contains as many cells as there are individuals and the observed proportions of subjects with disease in each cell must be 0 out of 1 or 1 out of 1. This can occur when at least one of the independent variables is continuous, but of course can also be simply a consequence of the way the data are input. It is possible that each individual is unique and we may not wish to group them.

If the data are in the form of tables most computer packages will provide a separate set of commands to carry out an analysis. Preserving the individual cases leads to the same regression estimates and allows for a more flexible analysis. This is discussed further in section 3.3.

Recall from Swinscow[1] that the purpose of statistical analysis is to take *samples* to estimate *population* parameters. In logistic regression we model the population parameters. If we consider the categorical grouped case first, denote the population probability of an event for a cell i by π_i. This is also called the "expected" value. Thus for an unbiased coin the population or expected probability for a "head" is 0.5. The dependent variable y_i is the observed proportion of events in the cell (say the proportion of heads in a set of tosses) and we write $E(y_i) = \pi_i$ where E denotes "expected value". Also recall that if an event has probability π_i, then the *odds* for that event are $\pi_i/(1 - \pi_i)$ to 1. Thus the *odds* of a head to a tail are 1 to 1.

The model is

$$\log_e\{\pi_i/(1 - \pi_i)\} = \text{logit}(\pi_i) = \beta_0 + \beta_1 X_{i1} + \ldots + \beta_p X_{ip}. \quad (3.1)$$

where the independent variables are $X_{i1}, \ldots, X_{ip}$.

The term on the left-hand side of the equation is the log odds of success, and is often called the *logistic* or *logit* transform.

The reason why model (3.1) is useful is that the coefficients β are related to the *odds ratio* in 2×2 tables. Suppose we had only one covariate x, which was binary and simply takes the values 0 or 1. Then the *odds ratio* associated with x and y is given by $\exp(\beta)$ (note *not* "relative risk" as is sometimes stated). If x is continuous then $\exp(\beta)$ is the odds ratio associated with a unit increase in x.

The main justification for the logit transformation is that the odds ratio is a natural parameter to use for binary outcomes, and the logit transformation relates this to the independent variables in a convenient manner. It can also be justified as follows. The right-hand side of equation (3.1) is potentially unbounded, that is can range from minus to plus ∞. On the left-hand side, a probability must lie between 0 and 1. An odds ratio must lie between 0 and ∞. A log odds ratio, or logit, is unbounded and has the same potential range as the right-hand side of equation (3.1).

Note at this stage that the *observed* values of the dependent variable are not in the equation. They are linked to the model by the Binomial distribution (described in Appendix 2). Thus in cell i if we observe y_i successes in n_i subjects, we assume that the y_i are distributed Binomially with probability π_i. The parameters in the model are estimated by maximum likelihood, also discussed in Appendix 2. Of course we do not know the population values π_i, and in the modelling process we substitute into the model the estimated or fitted values.

Often, by analogy to multiple regression, the model is described in the literature as above, but with the observed proportion, p_i, replacing π_i. This misses out on the second part of a model, the error distribution which links the two. One could, in fact, use the observed proportions and fit the model by least squares as in multiple regression. In the cases where p_i is not close to 0 or 1, this will often do well, although the interpretation of the model is different to that of equation (3.1) because the link with odds ratios is missing. With modern computers the method of maximum likelihood is easy and is to be preferred. When the dependent variable is 0/1, the logit of the dependent variable does not exist. This may lead some people to believe that logistic regression is impossible in these circumstances. However, as explained earlier the model uses the logit of the *expected* value, not the observed value, and the model ensures the expected value is greater than 0 and less than 1.

We may wish to calculate the probability of an event. Suppose we have estimated the coefficients in equation (3.1) to be $b_0, b_1, ..., b_p$. As in Chapter 1 we write the estimated linear predictor as

$$\text{LP}_i = b_0 + b_1 X_{i1} + ... + b_p X_{ip}$$

Then equation (3.1) can be written as

$$\hat{\pi}_i = \frac{e^{LP_i}}{1+e^{LP_i}} \tag{3.2}$$

where $\hat{\pi}_i$ is an estimate of π_i and estimates the probability of an event from the model. These are the predicted or fitted values for y_i. A good model will give predictions $\hat{\pi}_i$ close to the observed proportions y_i/n_i.

Further details of logistic regression are given in Collett[2] and Hosmer and Lemeshow.[3]

3.2 Uses of logistic regression

1. As a substitute for multiple regression when the outcome variable is binary in cross-sectional and cohort studies and in clinical trials. Thus we would use logistic regression to investigate the relationship between a causal variable and a binary output variable, allowing for confounding variables which can be categorical or continuous.

2. As a discriminant analysis, to try and find factors that discriminate two groups. Here the outcome would be a binary variable indicating membership to a group. For example one might want to discriminate men and women on psychological test results.

3. To develop prognostic indicators, such as the risk of complications from surgery.

4. To analyse case-control studies and matched case-control studies.

3.3 Interpreting a computer output: grouped analysis

Most computer packages have different procedures for the situations when the data appear in a grouped table, and when they refer to individuals. It is usually easier to store data on an individual basis, since it can be used for a variety of purposes. However, when the dependent variables are all categorical, the coefficients and standard errors of a logistic regression analysis will be exactly the same for the grouped procedure, where the dependent variable is the number of successes in the group and for the ungrouped procedure where the dependent variable is simply 0/1. In general it is easier to examine the goodness of fit of the model in the grouped case.

Consider the example of given in Swinscow[1] in which the association between breast and bottle feeding at 3 months was examined for printers' and farmers' wives. We can define an event as a baby being breast fed for 3 months or more and we have a single categorical variable X_1 which takes the value 1 if the mother were a farmer's wife and 0 if she were a printer's wife. The data are given in Table 3.1.

Table 3.1 Numbers of wives of printers and farmers who breast fed their babies for less than 3 months or for 3 months or more (from Swinscow Table 8.3)[1]

Wife	< 3months	≥ 3months	Total
Printers' wives	36	14	50
Farmers' wives	30	25	55
Total	66	39	105

We can rewrite this for the computer either as for a grouped analysis:

Y	n	Occupation (1 = printer, 0 = farmer)
36	50	1
30	55	0

or as the following for an ungrouped analysis:

Y (breast feeding) (1 for <3 months, 0 for ≥3 months)	Occupation (1=printer, 0 = farmer)
1 (36 times)	1
1 (30 times)	0
0 (14 times)	1
0 (25 times)	0

Table 3.2 Output from a logistic regression program using data in Table 3.1

Logit estimates

				Number of obs =	105
				LR chi2(0) =	0.00
				Prob > chi2 =	.
Log likelihood = −69.26972 | | | | Pseudo R2 = | 0.0000 |

_outcome	Coef.	Std. Err.	z	P>|z|	[95% Conf. Interval]
_cons	.5260931	.2019716	2.605	0.009	.130236 .9219502

.

Logit estimates

				Number of obs =	105
				LR chi2(1) =	3.45
				Prob > chi2 =	0.0631
Log likelihood = −67.543174 | | | | Pseudo R2 = | 0.0249 |

breast	Coef.	Std. Err.	z	P>|z|	[95% Conf. Interval]
Occupatn	−.7621401	.415379	−1.835	0.067	−1.576268 .0519878
_cons	.9444616	.3149704	2.999	0.003	.327131 1.561792

breast	Odds Ratio	Std. Err.	z	P>|z|	[95% Conf. Interval]
Occupatn	.4666667	.1938435	−1.835	0.067	.2067453 1.053363

The output for a logistic regression for these data (in the second form) is shown in Table 3.2. The first section gives the fit for a constant term and the second the fit of the term occupation. The output can be requested in terms of either the coefficients in the model, or the odds ratios and here we give both. The output also gives the log-likelihood values, which are described in Appendix 2, and can be thought of as a sort of residual sum of squares.

The log-likelihood for the model without the occupation term is −69.27 and with the occupation term is −67.54. The difference, multiplied by −2 is the "LR chi2(1)" term (LR for likelihood ratio), which is 3.45. This can be interpreted as a chi-squared statistic with 1 degree of freedom. This is further described in Appendix 2. It can be seen that the likelihood ratio chi-squared statistic for this model has 1 degree of freedom, since it has only one term (occupation), and is not significant (P =0.0631).

The "pseudo R2" is described in Appendix 2 and is based on the proportionate drop in the log-likelihood. It is analogous to the R^2

term in linear regression which gives the proportion of variance accounted for by the model. This is less easy to interpret in the binary case, and it is suggested that one considers only the rough magnitude of the pseudo R2. In this case a value of 0.0249 implies that the model does not fit particularly well since only a small proportion of the variance is accounted for.

The Wald statistic, which is the ratio of the estimate b to its standard error, i.e. $z = b/SE(b) = (-0.7621/0.4154) = -1.85$. The square of this, 3.3665, is close to the likelihood ratio statistic, and the corresponding P value (0.067) is close to the LR chi-squared value.

The conventional chi-squared statistic, described in Swinscow[1] is neither the Wald nor the likelihood ratio and is in fact the third of the statistics derived from likelihood theory, the score statistic (see Appendix 2). This has value 3.418, and is very close to the other two statistics.

If b_1 is the estimate of β_1 then $\exp(b_1)$ is the estimated odds ratio associated with X_1. The odds ratio associated with Table 3.1 is given by $(30 \times 14)/(36 \times 25) = 0.4667$. This figure also appears in the computer output given in Table 3.2. The coefficient in the model is -0.7621, and the odds ratio (OR) is given by $\exp(-0.7621) = 0.4667$. Thus printers' wives are nearly half as likely to breast feed for 3 months or more than farmers' wives.

A 95% confidence interval for β (which is a log odds) is given by $b \pm 1.96 \times SE(b)$. This is sometimes known as a *Wald confidence interval* (see section 3.4) since it is based on the Wald test. Thus a 95% confidence interval for the odds ratio is $\exp\{b - 1.96 \times SE(b)\}$ to $\exp\{b + 1.96 \times SE(b)\}$. This is asymmetric about OR, in contrast to the confidence intervals in linear regression. For example, from Table 3.2, the confidence interval for the estimate is $\exp(-0.7621 - 1.96 \times 0.4154)$ to $\exp(-0.7621 + 1.96 \times 0.4154)$ or 0.207 to 1.053, which is asymmetric about 0.4667. Note the confidence interval includes one, which is to be expected since the significance test is non-significant at $P = 0.05$. In general this will hold true, but there can be slight discrepancies with the significance test especially if the odds ratio is large because the test of significance may be based on the likelihood ratio test or the score test whereas the confidence interval is usually based on the Wald test.

3.4 Logistic regression in action

Lavie *et al.*[4] surveyed 2677 adults referred to a sleep clinic with suspected sleep apnoea. They developed an apnoea severity index, and related this to the presence or absence of hypertension.

The questions that they wished to answer are:

(i) Is the apnoea index predictive of hypertension, allowing for age, sex and body mass index?

(ii) Is sex a predictor of hypertension, allowing for the other covariates?

The results are given in Table 3.3 and the authors chose to give the regression coefficients (log odds) and the Wald confidence interval.

Table 3.3 Risk factors for hypertension[4]

Risk factor	Estimate (log odds)	(Wald 95% CI)	Odds ratio
Age (10 years)	0.805	(0.718 to 0.892)	2.24
Sex (male)	0.161	(−0.061 to 0.383)	1.17
BMI (5 kg/m^2)	0.332	(0.256 to 0.409)	1.39
Apnoea index (10 units)	0.116	(0.075 to 0.156)	1.12

The coefficient associated with the dummy variable sex is 0.161, so the odds of having hypertension for a man are exp(0.161)=1.17 times that of a woman in this study. On the odds ratio scale the 95% confidence interval is exp(−0.061) to exp(0.383)=0.94 to 1.47. Note that this includes one (as we would expect since the confidence interval for the regression coefficient includes zero) and so we cannot say that sex is a significant predictor of hypertension in this study. We interpret the age coefficient by saying that, if we had two people of the same sex, and given that their BMI and apnoea index were also the same, but one subject was 10 years older than the other, then we would predict that the older subject would be 2.24 times more likely to have hypertension. The reason for the choice of 10 years is because that is how age was scaled. Note that factors that are additive on the log scale are multiplicative on the odds scale. Thus a man who is ten years older than a woman is predicted to be 2.24×1.17=2.62 times more likely to have hypertension. Thus the model assumes that age and sex act independently on hypertension, and so the risks multiply. This can be checked by including an interaction term between age and sex in the model as described in Chapter 2. If this is found to be significant, it implies there is *effect modification* between age and sex, and so if the interaction was positive it would imply that an older man is at much greater risk of hypertension than would be predicted by his age and sex separately.

3.5 Model checking

There are a number of ways the model may fail to describe the data well. Some of these are the same as those discussed in section 2.7 for linear regression, such as linearity of the coefficients in the linear predictor, influential observations and lack of an important confounder. It is easy to imagine the effect on a regression coefficient of deleting an individual observation, and it is important also to look for observations whose removal has a large influence on the model coefficients. These influential points are handled in logistic regression in a similar way to that described for multiple regression in Chapter 2. Some computer packages will give measures of influence for individuals in logistic regression.

Defining residuals is more difficult in logistic regression and model checking is different to the linear regression situation. Outlying observations can be difficult to check when the outcome variable has only two values 0 or 1. Further details are given by Collett[2] and Campbell.[5]

Issues particularly pertinent to logistic regression are: lack of fit; "extra-Binomial" variation; the logistic transform.

Lack of fit

If the independent variables are all categorical, then one can compare the observed proportions in each of the cells and those predicted by the model. However, if some of the input variables are continuous, one has to group the predicted values in some way. Hosmer and Lemeshow[3] suggest a number of methods. One suggestion is to group the predicted probabilities from the model π_i into tenths (by deciles), and compute the predicted number of successes between each decile as the sum of the predicted probabilities for those individuals in that group. The observed number of successes and failures can be compared using a chi-squared distribution with 8 degrees of freedom[1] (Chapter 5). A well-fitting model should be able to predict the observed successes and failures in each group with some accuracy. A significant chi-squared value indicates that the model is a poor description of the data.

"Extra-Binomial" variation

Unlike multiple regression, where the size of the residual variance is not specified in advance and is estimated from the data, in logistic regression a consequence of the Binomial model is that the residual variance is predetermined. However, the value specified by the model may be less (and sometimes greater) than that observed, and is known as "extra-Binomial variation". When the variance is greater than expected it is known as "overdispersion" and it can occur when the data are not strictly independent. For example, repeated outcomes within an individual, or patients grouped by general practitioner. Whilst the estimate of the regression coefficients is not unduly affected, the estimates of the standard errors are usually underestimated, leading to confidence intervals that are too narrow. In the past this has been dealt with by an approximate method, for example by scaling the standard errors upwards to allow for the underestimation, but not changing the estimates of the coefficients. However, this situation is now viewed as a special case of what is known as a *random effects model* in which one (or more) of the regression coefficients β is regarded as random with a mean and variance that can be estimated, rather than fixed. This will be described in Chapter 5.

The logistic transform is inappropriate

The logistic transform is not the only one that converts a probability ranging from 0 to 1 to a variable that potentially can range from minus infinity to plus infinity. Other examples are the *probit* and the *complementary log–log* transform given by $\log(-\log(1-\pi))$. The latter is useful when events (such as deaths) occur during a cohort study and leads to survival analyses (see Chapter 4). Some packages enable one to use different link functions and usually they will give similar results. The logistic link is the easiest to interpret and the one generally recommended.

3.6 Interpreting a computer output: ungrouped analysis

A consecutive series of 170 patients were scored for risk of complications following abdominal operations with an APACHE risk score (C. Johnston, personal communication). Their weight (in kilograms) was also measured. The outcome was whether the complications after the operation were mild or severe. The output is given in Table 3.4. Here the coefficients are expressed as odds ratios. The interpretation of the model is that, *for a fixed weight,* a subject who scores one unit higher on the APACHE will have an increased odds ratio of severe complications of 1.9 and this is highly significant ($P < 0.001$).

Table 3.4 Output from a logistic regression on data from abdominal operations (Johnston, personal communication)

Logit estimates				Number of obs	=	170
				LR chi2(2)	=	107.01
				Prob > chi2	=	0.0000
Log likelihood = −56.866612				Pseudo R2	=	0.4848

severity	Odds Ratio	Std. Err.	z	P>|z|	[95% Conf. Interval]	
apache	1.898479	.2008133	6.060	0.000	1.543012	2.335836
weight	1.039551	.0148739	2.711	0.007	1.010804	1.069116

Logistic model for severity, goodness of fit test
(Table collapsed on quantiles of estimated probabilities)

number of observations	=	170
number of groups	=	10
Hosmer-Lemeshow chi2(8)	=	4.94
Prob > chi2	=	0.7639

As an illustration of whether the model is a good fit, we see the Hosmer–Lemeshow statistic discussed above is not significant, indicating that the observed counts and those predicted by the model are quite close, and thus the model describes the data reasonably well. In practice, investigators use the Hosmer–Lemeshow statistic to reassure themselves that the model describes the data and so they can interpret the coefficients. However, one can object to the idea of using a significance test to determine goodness of fit, before using another test to determine whether coefficients are significant. If the first test is not significant, it does not tell us that the model is true, only that we do not have enough evidence to reject it. Since no model is exactly true, with enough data the goodness of fit test will always reject the model. However the model may be "good enough" for a valid analysis. If the model does not fit, is it valid to make inferences from the model? In general the answer is "yes", but care is needed!

A further check on the model is to look at the influential points and these are available in many packages now. In STATA an overall influential statistic, labelled Pregibon's "dbeta" is available, but not influential statistics for each of the regression parameters as in multiple regression. A plot of the dbeta against the probability of severe complications is given in Figure 3.1 and indicates that there are about five observations that are influential on the coefficients of the model, and these could be explored in more detail.

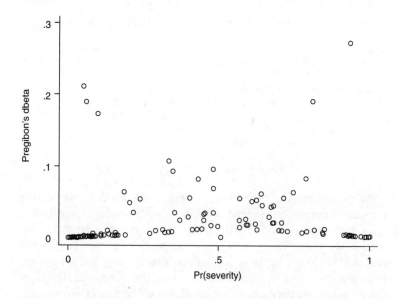

Figure 3.1 A plot of an influential statistic against estimated probability of an event for abdominal data (C. Johnston, personal communication).

Logit/logistic/log-linear

Readers of computer manuals may come across a different form of model known as a *log-linear model*. Log-linear models are used to analyse large contingency tables and can be used to analyse binary data instead of logistic regression. Some earlier computer programs only allowed log-linear models. However in general they are more difficult to interpret than logistic regression models. They differ from logistic models in that:

- There is no clear division between dependent and independent variables.

- In logistic regression the independent variables can be continuous.

- In log-linear models one has to include all the variables, dependent and independent into the model first. An association between a dependent and independent variable is measured by fitting an interaction term. Thus for a log-linear model, in the Lavie *et al.*[4] study example, one would first have to split age into groups, say "young" and "old" (since age is continuous). One would then have to fit parameters corresponding to the proportion of subjects with and without hypertension and who are in the old or young age group before fitting a parameter corresponding to the interaction between the two to assess whether age and hypertension were associated. By contrast, in logistic regression, the presence or absence of hypertension is unequivocally the dependent variable and age an independent variable.

3.7 Case–control studies

One of the main uses of logistic regression is in the analysis of case-control studies. In Swinscow[1] we saw that it was a happy fact that an odds ratio is reversible. Thus the odds ratio is the same whether we consider the odds of printers' wives being more likely to breast feed for more than 3 months than farmers' wives, or the odds of those who breast feed for more than 3 months being more likely to be printers' wives than farmers' wives. This reversal of logic occurs in case-control studies, where we select cases with a disease and controls without the disease. We then investigate the amount of exposure to a suspected cause that each has had. This is in contrast to a cohort study, where we consider those exposed or not exposed to a suspected cause, and then follow them up for disease development.

If we employ logistic regression and code the dependent variable as 1 if the subject is a case and 0 for a control, then the estimates of the coefficients associated with exposure are the log odds ratios, which, provided the disease is relatively rare, will provide valid estimates of the relative risk for the exposure variable.

3.8 Interpreting a computer output: unmatched case-control study

Consider the meta-analysis of four case control studies described in Altman et al.[6] from Wald et al.[7] (1986).

Table 3.5 Exposure to passive smoking among female lung cancer cases and controls in four studies.[7]

Study	Lung cancer cases		Controls		Odds ratio
	Exposed	Unexposed	Exposed	Unexposed	
1	14	8	61	72	2.07
2	33	8	164	32	0.80
3	13	11	15	10	0.79
4	91	43	254	148	1.23

For the computer this is rewritten:

Y (cases)	n (cases+controls)	Exposed	Study
14	75	1	1
8	80	0	1
33	197	1	2
etc.			

In the above table there are eight rows, being the number of unique study × exposure combinations. The dependent variable for the model is the number of cases. One also has to specify the total number of cases and controls for each row. The output from a logistic regression program is given in Table 3.6. Here *study* is a four level categorical variable, which is a confounder and modelled with three dummy variables as described in Chapter 2. This is known as a *fixed effects* analysis. Chapter 5 gives a further discussion on the use of dummy variables in cases such as these. The program gives the option of getting the output as the log odds (the regression coefficients) or the odds ratio. The main result is that lung cancer and passive smoking are associated with an odds ratio of 1.198, with 95% CI 0.858 to 1.672. The pseudo R2 which is automatically given by STATA is difficult to interpret and should not be quoted. It is printed automatically and illustrates one of the hazards of reading routine output.

Table 3.6 Output from a logistic regression program for the case-control study in Table 3.3.

Logit estimates		Number of obs	=	977
		LR chi2(4)	=	30.15
		Prob > chi2	=	0.0000
Log likelihood = −507.27463		Pseudo R2	=	0.0289

_outcome	Coef.	Std. Err.	z	P>|z|	[95% Conf.	Interval]
Istudy_2	.1735811	.292785	0.593	0.553	−.4002669	.7474292
Istudy_3	1.74551	.3673518	4.752	0.000	1.025514	2.465506
Istudy_4	.6729274	.252246	2.668	0.008	.1785343	1.16732
exposed	.1802584	.1703595	1.058	0.290	−.1536401	.5141569
_cons	−1.889435	.2464887	−7.665	0.000	−2.372544	−1.406326

_outcome	Odds Ratio	Std. Err.	z	P>|z|	[95% Conf.	Interval]
Istudy_2	1.189557	.3482845	0.593	0.553	.6701412	2.111565
Istudy_3	5.728823	2.104494	4.752	0.000	2.788528	11.76944
Istudy_4	1.959967	.4943937	2.668	0.008	1.195464	3.213371
exposed	1.197527	.2040101	1.058	0.290	.8575806	1.672228

3.9 Matched case-control studies

In matched case-control studies each case is matched directly with one or more controls. For a valid analysis the matching should be taken into account. An obvious method would be to fit dummy variables as strata for each of the matched groups. However, it can be shown[8] that this will produce biased estimates. Instead we use a

51

method known as *conditional logistic regression*. In a simple 2×2 table this gives a result equivalent to a McNemar test.[1] It is a flexible method, that with most modern software allows cases to have differing numbers of controls; it is not required to have exact 1:1 matching.

The logic for a *conditional* likelihood is quite complex, but the argument can be simplified. Suppose in a matched case–control study with exactly one control per case we had a logistic model such as equation (3.1), and for pair i the probability of an event for the case was π_{i0} and for the control π_{i1}. Given that we know that one of the pair *must* be the case, i.e. there must be one and only one event in the pair, *conditional* on the pair, the probability of the event for the case is simply $\pi_{i0}/(\pi_{i0}+\pi_{i1})$. As an example, suppose you knew that a husband and wife team had won a lottery, and the husband had bought five tickets and the wife one. Then if you were asked the probability that the husband had won the lottery, he would be five times more likely than his wife, i.e. a conditional probability of 5/6 relative to 1/6. We can form a conditional likelihood by multiplying the probabilities for each case-control pair, and maximise it in a manner similar to that for ordinary logistic regression and this is now simply achieved with many computer packages.

The model is the same as equation (3.1), but the method of estimating the parameters is different, using conditional likelihood rather than unconditional likelihood. As discussed more extensively in Swinscow[1] any factor which is the same in the case-control set, for example a matching factor, cannot appear as an independent variable in the model.

3.10 Interpreting a computer output: matched case-control study

These data are taken from Eason *et al.*[9] and described in Altman *et al.*[6] Thirty-five patients who died in hospital from asthma were individually matched for sex and age with 35 control subjects who had been discharged from the same hospital in the preceding year. The adequacy of monitoring of the patients was independently assessed and the results given in Table 3.7.

For a computer analysis this may be written as a datafile with

35×2=70 rows, one for each case and control as shown in Table 3.8. For example the first block refers to the 10 deaths and 10 survivors for whom monitoring is inadequate.

Table 3.7 Adequacy of monitoring in hospital of 35 deaths and matched survivors with asthma.[9]

		Deaths	
		Inadequate	Adequate
Survivors (controls)	Inadequate	10	3
	Adequate	13	9

Table 3.8 Data from Table 3.7 written for a computer analysis using conditional logistic regression.

Pair number	Case/control(1=death)	Monitoring (1=inadequate)
1	1	1
1	0	1
2	1	1
2	0	1
(for 10 pairs)		
11	1	1
11	0	0
12	1	1
12	0	0
(for 13 pairs)		
24	1	0
24	0	1
(for 3 pairs)		
28	1	0
28	0	0
(for 9 pairs)		

The logic for conditional logistic regression is the same as for McNemar's test. When the monitoring is the same for both case and control, the pair do not contribute to the estimate of the odds ratio. It is only when they differ that we can calculate an odds ratio.

From Table 3.7, the estimated odds ratio of dying in hospital associated with inadequate monitoring is given by the ratio of the numbers of the two discordant pairs, namely 13/3=4.33.

Table 3.9 Output from conditional logistic regression of the matched case-control study in Table 3.8.

Conditional (fixed-effects) logistic regression   Number of obs = 70

	LR chi2(1) = 6.74
	Prob > chi2 = 0.0094
Log likelihood = −20.891037	Pseudo R2 = 0.1389

deaths	Odds Ratio	Std. Err.	z	P>|z|	[95% Conf. Interval]
monitor	4.333333	2.775524	2.289	0.022	1.234874 15.20623

The results of the conditional logistic regression are given in Table 3.9.

The P value for the Wald test is given as P=0.022, which is significant, suggesting that inadequate monitoring increases the risk of death. The P value for the likelihood ratio is 0.0094. Note the disparity between the likelihood ratio test and the Wald test P values. This is because the numbers in the table are small and the distribution discrete and so the approximations that all the methods use are less accurate. The McNemar's chi-square (a score test) is $(13-3)^2/(13+3)=6.25$ with P=0.012, which is mid-way between the likelihood ratio and the Wald test. Each value can be regarded as valid, and in cases of differences it is important to state which test was used for obtaining the P value and perhaps quote more than one. This is in contrast to linear regression in Chapter 2, where the three methods will all coincide.

The odds ratio is estimated as 4.33 with 95% confidence interval 1.23 to 15.21. This confidence interval differs somewhat from the confidence interval given in Altman *et al.*[6], p. 66 because an exact method was used there, which is preferable with small numbers.

Note that the advantage of conditional logistic regression over a simple McNemar test is that other covariates could be easily incorporated into the model. In the above example, we might also have measured the use of bronchodilators for all 70 subjects, as a risk factor for dying in hospital.

3.11 Conditional logistic regression in action

Churchill *et al.*[10] used a matched case-control study in which the cases were teenagers who had become pregnant over a three-year period. Three age-matched controls, closest in age to the case, who had no recorded teenage pregnancy were identified from within the same practice. The results were analysed by conditional logistic regression and showed that cases were more likely to have consulted in the year before conception than controls (odds ratio 2.70, 95% CI 1.56 to 4.66).

3.12 Reporting the results of logistic regression

- Summarise the logistic regression to include the number of observations in the analysis, the coefficient of the explanatory variable with its standard error and/or the odds ratio and the 95% confidence interval for the odds ratio and the P value.

- If a predictor variable is continuous, then it is often helpful to scale it to ease interpretation. For example, it is easier to think of the increased risk of death every 10 years, than the increased risk per year, which will be very close to 1.

- Specify which type of P value is quoted (e.g. likelihood ratio or Wald).

- Confirm that the assumptions for the logistic regression were met, in particular that the events are independent and the relationship plausibly log-linear. If the design is a matched one, ensure that the analysis uses an appropriate method such as conditional logistic regression.

- Report any sensitivity analysis carried out.

- Name the statistical package used in the analysis. This is important because different packages sometimes have different definitions of common terms.

- Specify whether the explanatory variables were tested for interaction.

3.13 Reading about logistic regression

In addition to the points in sections 1.11 and 2.10.

- Is logistic regression appropriate? Is the outcome a simple binary variable? If there is a time attached to the outcome then survival analysis might be better (Chapter 4).

- The outcome is often described as "relative risks". Whilst this is often approximately true, they are better described as "approximate relative risks", or better "odds ratios". Note that for an odds ratio, a non-significant result is associated with a 95% confidence interval that includes one (not zero as in multiple regression).

- Have any sensitivity tests been carried out? Is there evidence of overdispersion?

- If the design is a matched case-control study, has conditional logistic regression been carried out?

Frequently asked questions

1. Does it matter how the independent variable is coded?
This depends on the computer package. Some packages will assume that any positive number is an event and zero is a non-event. Changing the code from 0/1 to 1/0 will simply change the sign of the coefficient in the regression model.

2. How is the odds ratio associated with a continuous variable interpreted?
The odds ratio associated with a continuous variable is the ratio of odds of an event in two subjects, in which one subject is one unit higher than another. This assumes a linear model which can be hard to validate. One suggestion is to divide the data into five approximately equal groups, ordered on the continuous variable. Fit a model with four dummy variables corresponding to the four higher groups, with the lowest fifth as baseline. Look at the *coefficients* in the model (*not* the odds ratios). If they are plausibly increasing linearly then a linear model may be reasonable. Otherwise report the results of the model using the dummy variables.

Multiple choice questions

1. An unmatched case-control study looking at breast cancer and the oral contraceptive pill included smoking habit (yes/no) as a potential confounder. The odds ratio of breast cancer amongst ever pill-takers was 1.5 (95% CI 1.1 to 2.0) unadjusted and 1.2 (95% CI 0.9 to 1.5) adjusted.

(i) The result allowing for smoking is statistically significant.
(ii) It is important to allow for smoking in the analysis.
(iii) The women are matched for smoking habit.
(iv) The approximate relative risk for breast cancer in a non-smoking woman who has taken the oral contraceptive pill is 1.2.
(v) The dependent variable in the model is whether or not a woman has breast cancer.

2. Consider a case–control study of suicide in psychiatric patients, in which the cases were matched by age and sex to alive controls. The study wished to look at the effect of continuity of care (a binary variable) on suicide risk. The coefficient in the appropriate model for a breakdown in continuity of care was 2.

(i) The correct analysis is conditional logistic regression.
(ii) One cannot include age in the model as an independent variable.
(iii) The odds ratio of suicide for a breakdown of continuity of care is $\exp(2) = 7.4$.
(iv) It is important to have exactly the same number of controls as cases.
(v) An ordinary logistic regression will give very different results to a conditional logistic regression.

References

1 Swinscow TDV. *Statistics at Square One, 9th edn.* (revised by MJ Campbell). London: BMJ Books, 1996.
2 Collett D. *Modelling Binary Data.* London: Chapman and Hall, 1991.
3 Hosmer DW, Lemeshow S. *Applied Logistic Regression.* New York: John Wiley, 1989.

4 Lavie P, Herer P, Hoffstein V. Obstructive sleep apnoea syndrome as a risk factor for hypertension: population study. *BMJ* 2000; **320**: 479–82.

5 Campbell MJ. Teaching logistic regression. In: Pereira-Mendoza L, Kea LS, Kee TW, Wong W-K, eds. *Statistical Education-expanding the Network. Proceedings of the fifth international conference on teaching statistics.* Voorburg: 1S1 1998: 281–6.

6 Altman DG, Machin D, Bryant TN, Gardner MJ, eds. *Statistics with Confidence.* London: BMJ Books, 2000.

7 Wald NJ, Nanchahal K, Thompson SG, Cuckle HS. Does breathing other people's tobacco smoke cause lung cancer? *BMJ* 1986; **293**: 1217–22.

8 Breslow NE, Day NE. *Statistical Methods in Cancer Research 1: The analysis of case control studies.* Lyon: IARC, 1980.

9 Eason J, Markowe HLJ. Controlled investigation of deaths from asthma in hospitals in the North East Thames region. *BMJ* 1987; **294**, 1255–8.

10 Churchill D, Allen J, Pringle M, Hippisley-Cox J, Ebdon D, Macpherson M and Bradley S. Consultation patterns and provision of contraception in general practice before teenage pregnancy: case control study. *BMJ* 2000; **321:** 486–9.

4 Survival analysis

Summary

When the dependent variable is a survival time, we can use a model known as a *proportional hazard model*, also referred to as a *Cox model*. In Swinscow[1] we described the log-rank test, which is appropriate for a single, binary, independent variable. The Cox proportional hazard model is a generalisation of this to allow for multiple independent variables which can be binary, categorical and continuous.

4.1 Introduction

In Swinscow[1] we discussed survival analysis, in which the key variable is the time until some event. Commonly it is the time from treatment for a disease to death, but in fact it can be time to any event. Examples include time for a fracture to heal and time that a nitroglycerine patch stays in place. As for binary outcomes, we imagine individuals suffering an *event*, but attached to this *event* is a *survival time*.

There are two main distinguishing features about survival analysis.

- The presence of *censored observations*. These can arise in two ways. Firstly, individuals can be removed from the data set, without suffering an event. For example in a study looking at survival from some disease, they may be lost to follow up, or get run over by a bus and so all we know is that they survived up to a particular point in time. Secondly, the study might be closed at a particular time point, as for example when a clinical trial is halted. Those still in the study are also regarded as censored, since they were alive when data collection was stopped. Clinical trials often recruit over a period of time, so subjects recruited more recently will have less time to suffer an event than subjects recruited early on.

- The development of models that do not require a particular distribution for the survival times, so-called *semi-parametric models*. This methodology allows a great deal of flexibility, with fewer assumptions than are required for fully parametric models.

A critical assumption in these models is that the probability that an individual is censored is unrelated to the probability that the individual suffers an event. If individuals who respond poorly to a treatment are removed before death and treated as censored observations then the models that follow are invalid. This is the so-called *uninformative* or *non-informative censoring* assumption.

The important benefit of survival analysis over logistic regression, say, is that the time an individual spent in the study can be used in the analysis, even if they did not suffer an event. In survival, the fact that one individual spent only 10 days in the study, whereas another spent 10 years is taken into account. In contrast in a simple chi-squared test or in logistic regression, all that is analysed is whether the individual suffered an event or not.

Further details are given in Collett[2] and Parmar and Machin.[3]

4.2 The model

The dependent variable in survival analysis is what is known as the *hazard*. This is a probability of dying at a point in time, but it is conditional on surviving up to that point in time, which is why it is given a specific name.

Suppose we followed a cohort of 1000 people from birth to death. Say for the age group 45–54, there were 19 deaths. In a 10–year age group there are 10×1000 *person-years at risk*. We could think of the death rate per person-year for 45–54 year olds as $19/(10 \times 1000) = 1.9$ per 1000. However if there were only 910 people alive by the time they reached 45, then the risk of death per person-year in the next 10 years, having survived to 45 is $19/(10 \times 910) = 2.1$ per 1000 per year. This is commonly called the *force of mortality*. In general, suppose X people were alive at the start of a year in a particular age group, and x people died during a period of width t. The risk over that period is $x/(tX)$. If we imagine the width, t, of the interval getting narrower then the number of deaths x will also fall but the ratio x/t will stay constant. This gives us the *instantaneous death rate* or the *hazard rate* at a particular time. (An analogy might be measuring the speed of a car by measuring the time t it takes to cover a distance x from a particular point. By reducing x and t we get the instantaneous speed at a particular point.)

The model links the hazard to an individual i at time t, $h_i(t)$ to a baseline hazard $h_0(t)$ by

$$\text{Log}\{h_i(t)\}=\log\{h_0(t)\}+\beta_1 X_1+....+\beta_p X_p \qquad (4.1)$$

where x_1, x_p are covariates associated with individual i.

This can also be written as

$$h_i(t)=h_0(t)\exp(\beta_1 X_1+....+\beta_p X_p). \qquad (4.2)$$

The baseline hazard $h_0(t)$ serves as a reference point, and can be thought of as an intercept β_0 in multiple regression equation (2.1). The important difference here is that it changes with time, whereas the intercept in multiple regression is constant. Similar to the intercept term, the hazard $h_0(t)$ in equation (4.1) represents the death rate for an individual whose covariates are all zero, which may be misleading if, say, age is a covariate. However it is not important that these values are realistic, but that they act as a reference for the individuals in the study.

Model (4.1) can be contrasted with model (3.1) which used the logit transform, rather than the log. Unlike model (3.1) which yields odds ratios, this model yields *relative risks*. Thus if we had one binary covariate X, then $\exp(\beta)$ is the relative risk of (say) death for $X=1$ compared to $X=0$. Model (4.1) is used in *prospective studies*, where a relative risk can be measured.

This model was introduced by Cox[4] and is frequently referred to as the *Cox regression model*. It is called the *proportional hazards model* because if we imagine two individuals i and j, then equation (4.1) assumes that $h_i(t)/h_j(t)$ is constant over time, i.e. even though $h_0(t)$ may vary, the two hazards for individuals whose covariates do not change with time remain proportional to each other. Since we do not have to specify $h_0(t)$, which is the equivalent of specifying a distribution for an error term, but we have specified a model in equation (4.1) which contains parameters the model is sometimes described oxymoronically as *semi-parametric*.

Given a prospective study such as a clinical trial, imagine we chose at random an individual *who has suffered an event* and their survival time is T. For any time t the survival curve $S(t)$ is $P(T \geq t)$, that is the probability of a random individual surviving longer than t. If we assume there are no censored observations, then the estimate of $S(t)$ is just the proportion of subjects who survive longer than t. When some of the observations can be censored it is estimated by the *Kaplan-Meier survival curve* described in Swinscow.[1] For any particular time t the hazard is

$$h(t) = P(T=t)/P(T \geq t)$$

Suppose $S_0(t)$ is the baseline survival curve corresponding to a hazard $h_0(t)$, and $S_x(t)$ is the survival curve corresponding to an individual with covariates $X_1, ... X_p$. Then it can be shown that under model (4.1),

$$S_x(t) = S_0(t)^{\exp(\beta_1 X_1 + ... + \beta_p X_p)} \qquad (4.3)$$

This relationship is useful for checking the proportional hazards assumption as we will show later.

The two important summary statistics are the number of events, and the *person-years at risk*. There can only be one event per individual.

4.3 Uses of Cox regression

1. As a substitute for logistic regression when the dependent variable is a binary event, but where there is also information on the length of time to the event. This may be censored if the event does not occur.

2. To develop prognostic indicators for survival after operations, survival from disease or time to other events, such as time to heal a fracture.

4.4 Interpreting a computer output

The method of fitting model (4.1) is again a form of maximum likelihood, known as *partial likelihood*. In this case the method is quite similar to the matched case-control approach described in Chapter 3. Thus one can consider any time at which an event has occurred, one individual (the case) has died and the remaining survivors are the controls. From model (4.1) one can write the probability that this particular individual is a case, given his/her covariates, compared to all the other survivors, and we attempt to find the coefficients that maximise this probability, for all the cases. Once again the computer output consists of the likelihood, the regression coefficients and their standard errors. Swinscow[1] describes data given by McIllmurray and Turkie[5] on the survival of 49 patients with Dukes' C colorectal cancer. The data are given in Table 4.1.

Table 4.1 Survival in 49 patients with Dukes' C colorectal cancer randomly assigned to either linolenic acid or control treatment (times with "+" are censored).

Treatment	Survival time (months)
γ-linolenic acid (n=25)	1+, 5+, 6, 6, 9+, 10, 10, 10+, 12, 12, 12, 12, 12+, 13+, 15+,16+, 20+, 24, 24+, 27+, 32, 34+, 36+, 36+, 44+
Control (n=24)	3+, 6, 6, 6, 6, 8, 8, 12, 12, 12+, 15+, 16+, 18+, 18+, 20, 22+, 24, 28+, 28+, 28+, 30, 30+, 33+, 42

The data are entered in the computer as:

Time	Event	Group (1=γ-linolenic acid, 0=control)
1	0	1
5	0	1
6	1	1
etc.		

The Kaplan–Meier survival curve is shown in Figure 4.1. Note the numbers at risk are shown on the graph. The output for the Cox regression is shown in Table 4.2

Ties in the data occur when two survival times are equal. There are a number of ways of dealing with these. The most common is known as *Breslow's method*, and this is an approximate method that will work well when there are not too many ties. Some packages will also allow an "exact" method, but this usually takes more computer time. An "exact" partial likelihood is shown here, because the large number of ties in the data may render approximate methods less accurate.

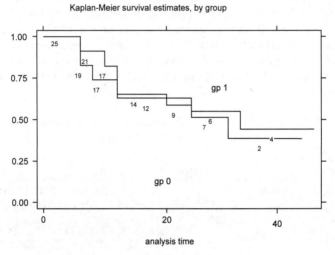

Figure 4.1 Kaplan–Meier survival curve for data in Table 4.1.

Ta.ble 4.2 Analysis of γ-linolenic acid data (computer output)

Cox regression – exact partial likelihood

No. of subjects	=	49	Number of obs =	49
No. of failures	=	22		
Time at risk	=	869		
			LR chi2(1) =	0.38
Log likelihood	=	−55.704161	Prob > chi2 =	0.5385

_t _d	Haz. Ratio	Std. Err.	z	P>|z|	[95% Conf. Interval]
gp	.7592211	.3407465	−0.614	0.539	.3150214 1.82977

From the output one can see that the hazard ratio associated with active treatment is 0.759 (95% CI 0.315 to 1.830). This has associated P values 0.54 by both the likelihood ratio and Wald methods, which implies there is little evidence of efficacy. The risk and confidence interval are very similar to those given in Swinscow,[1] chapter 12, which used the log-rank test. An important point to note is that the z statistic is *not* the ratio of the hazard ratio to its standard error, but rather the ratio of the *regression coefficient*, i.e. log (hazard ratio) to *its* standard error (which is not given in this output).

4.5 Survival analysis in action

Oddy *et al.*[6] looked at the association between breast feeding and developing asthma in a cohort of children to six years of age. The outcome was the age at developing asthma and they used Cox regression to examine the relationship with breast feeding and to adjust for confounding factors: sex, gestational age, being of Aboriginal descent and smoking in the household. They stated that "regression models were subjected to standard tests for goodness-of-fit including an investigation of the need for additional polynomial or interaction terms, an analysis of residuals, and tests of regression leverage and influence". They found that "other milk introduced before four months" was a risk factor for earlier asthma (hazard ratio 1.22, 95% CI 1.03 to 1.43, P=0.02).

4.6 Interpretation of the model

In the model (4.1), the predictor variables can be continuous or discrete. If there is just one binary predictor variable X, then the interpretation is closely related to the log-rank test described in Swinscow.[1] In this case, if the coefficient associated with X is b, then $\exp(b)$ is the *relative hazard* (often called the "relative risk") for individuals for whom $X=1$ compared with $X=0$. When there is more than one covariate, then the interpretations are very similar to those described in Chapter 3 for binary outcomes. In particular, since the linear predictor is related to the outcome by an exponential transform, what is additive in the linear predictor becomes multiplicative in the outcome, as in logistic regression section 3.4. In the asthma example the risk of asthma of 1.22 for children exposed to other milk products before four months assumes all other covariates are held constant. The model assumes multiplicative risks so that if the risk of developing asthma early is double in boys, then boys exposed to other milk products before four months will be at $2 \times 1.22 = 2.44$ times the risk of girls not exposed to milk products.

4.7 Generalisations of the model

Suppose Oddy et al.[6] did not wish to assume that the incidence rate for Aboriginal children was a constant multiple of the incidence rate of asthma for the non-Aboriginal children. Then we can fit two separate models to the two groups

$$\log(h_{iA}(t)) = \log(h_{0A}(t)) + \beta_1 X_1 + \dots + \beta_p X_p$$

for the aboriginal children and

$$\log(h_{iNA}(t)) = \log(h_{0NA}(t)) + \beta_1 X_1 + \dots + \beta_p X_p$$

for the non-aboriginal children. This is known as a *stratified Cox model*. Note that the regression coefficients, the βs, for the other covariates sex, gestational age and smoking in household are assumed to remain constant. This is an extension of the idea of fitting different intercepts for a categorical variable in multiple regression.

The model (4.1) assumes that the covariates are measured once at the beginning of the study. However, the model can be generalised to allow covariates to be time dependent. An example might be survival of a cohort of subjects exposed to asbestos, where a subject changes jobs over time and so changes his/her exposure to the dust. These are relatively easily incorporated into the computer analysis.

Another generalisation is to specify a distribution for $h_0(t)$ and use a fully parametric model. A common distribution is the *Weibull distribution*, which is a generalisation of the exponential distribution. This leads to what is known as an *accelerated failure time model*, so called because the effect of a covariate X is to change the time scale by a factor $\exp(-\beta)$. Thus rather than say a subject dies earlier, one may think of them as simply living faster! Details of this technique are beyond the scope of this book, but it is becoming widely available on computer packages. Usually it will give similar answers to the Cox regression model.

4.8 Model checking

The assumption about linearity of the model is similar to that in multiple regression modelling described in section 2.6 and can be checked in the same way. The methods for determining leverage and influence are also similar to those in multiple regression and so we refer the reader to section 2.7. There are a number of ways of calculating residuals, and various packages may produce some or all of *martingale residuals*, *Schoenfeld residuals* or *deviance residuals*. Details are beyond this book. However, since the Cox model is a semi-parametric model, the exact distribution of the residuals is unimportant. They can be used for checking outliers.

The new important assumption is that the hazard ratio remains constant over time. This is most straightforward when we have two groups to compare with no covariates. The simplest check is to plot the Kaplan–Meier survival curves for each group together. If they cross, then the proportional hazards assumption may be violated. For small data sets, where there may be a great deal of error attached to the survival curve, it is possible for curves to cross, even under the proportional hazards assumption. However, it should be clear that an overall test of whether one group has better survival than the other is meaningless when the answer will depend on the time that the test is made. A more sophisticated check is based on what is known as the *complementary log–log plot*. Suppose we have two groups with survival curves $S_1(t)$ and $S_2(t)$. We assume that the two groups are similar in all prognostic variables, except group membership. From equations (4.1) and (4.3), if the proportional hazard assumption holds true, then

$$\log\{-\log(S_1(t))\} = k + \log\{-\log(S_2(t))\}$$

where k is a constant. This implies that if we plot both $\log(-\log(S_1(t)))$ and $\log(-\log(S_2(t)))$ against t, then the two curves will be parallel, distance k apart.

This graph is plotted for the data in Table 4.2, and shown in Figure 4.2. It can be seen that the two curves overlap considerably, but there is no apparent divergence between them, and so they are plausibly parallel.

There are also a number of formal tests of proportional hazards and further details are given in Parmar and Machin (pp. 176–7).[3] Most packages will provide a number of such tests. As an example

Table 4.3 shows the result of a test of proportional hazards, based on the Schoenfeld residuals and given by STATA.[7] It can be seen that this agrees with the intuitive graphical test that there is little evidence of a lack of proportional hazards.

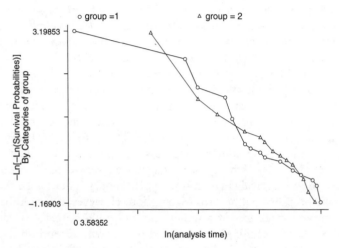

Figure 4.2 Log–log plot of survival curve in Figure 4.1.

Table 4.3 Test of proportional hazards assumption (computer output).

Time: Time

	chi2	df	Prob>chi2
global test	0.26	1	0.6096

The problems of testing proportional hazards are much more difficult when there are large numbers of covariates. In particular, it is assumed that the proportional hazards assumption remains true for one variable independent of all the other covariates. In practice, most of the covariates will simply be potential confounders, and it is questionable whether statistical inference is advanced by assiduously testing each for proportionality in the model. It is important, however that the main predictors, for example treatment group in a clinical trial, be tested for proportional hazards because it is impossible to interpret a fixed estimated relative risk if the true risk varies with time.

The other assumptions about the model are not testable from the data, but should be verified from the protocol. These include the fact that the events of being censored and suffering an event are independent. Thus in a survival study, one should ensure that patients are not removed from the study just before they die. Survival studies often recruit patients over a long period of time. It is also important that other factors remain constant over the period, such as the way patients are recruited into a study, and the diagnosis of the disease.

4.9 Reporting the results of a survival analysis

- Specify the nature of the censoring, and as far as possible validate that the censoring is non-informative.

- Report the total number of events, subjects and person-time of follow up, with some measure of variability such as a range for the latter. For a trial this should be done by treatment group.

- Report an estimated survival rate at a given time, by group, with confidence intervals.

- Display the Kaplan–Meier survival curves by group. To avoid misinterpretation of the right-hand end, terminate the curve when the number at risk is small, say five. It is often useful to show the numbers at risk at regular time intervals, as shown in Figure 4.1. For large studies this can be done at fixed time points, and shown just below the time axis.

- Specify the regression model used and note sensitivity analyses undertaken, and tests for proportionality of hazards.

- Specify a measure of risk for each explanatory variable, with a confidence interval and a precise P value. Note that these can be called relative risks, but it is perhaps better to refer to relative hazards.

- Report the computer program used for the analysis. Many papers just quote Cox[4] without much evidence of having read that paper!

4.10 Reading about the results of a survival analysis

- Is the proportional hazards assumption reasonable and has it been validated?

- Are the conclusions critically dependent on the assumptions?

- In trials, are numbers of censored observations given by treatment group?

Frequently asked question

Does it matter how the event variable is coded?

Unlike logistic regression, coding an event variable 1/0 instead of 0/1 has a major effect on the analysis. Thus it is vitally important to distinguish between the events (say deaths) and the censored times (say survivors). This is because, unlike odds ratios, hazard ratios are not symmetric to the coding and it matters if we are interested in survival or death. For example, if in two groups the mortality was 10% and 15% respectively, we would say that the second group has a 50% increased mortality. However, the survival rates in the two groups are 90% and 85% respectively, and so the second group has a 5/90=6% reduced survival rate.

Exercise

The table at the end of this chapter is an analysis of some data given by Piantadosi.[8] It concerns survival of 76 patients with mesothelioma, and potential prognostic variables are age (yrs), sex, weight change (wtchg), performance status (ps) (high or low) and five histologic subtypes. The analysis has been stratified by performance status, because it was felt that this may not have proportional hazards. Two models were fitted. One with age, sex and weight change, and the second including histologic status as a set of dummy variables. The purpose of the analysis was to find significant prognostic factors for survival.

Fill in the missing values in the output (A to G)

Model 1

Iteration 0: log likelihood = 188.55165

Stratified Cox regr. −Breslow method for ties

No. of subjects	=	76	Number of obs	=	76
No. of failures	=	63			
Time at risk	=	32380			
			LR chi2(A)	=	B
Log likelihood	= −188.04719		Prob > chi2	=	0.7991

_t _d	Coef.	Std. Err.	z	P>|z|	[95% Conf. Interval]	
age	.0038245	.0128157	0.298	0.765	−.0212939	.0289429
wtchg	.2859577	.3267412	0.875	0.381	−.3544433	.9263586
sex	−.1512113	.3102158	C	0.626	D	E

Stratified by ps

_t _d	Haz. Ratio	Std. Err.	z	P>|z|	[95% Conf. Interval]	
age	1.003832	.0128648	0.298	0.765	.9789312	1.029366
wtchg	1.331036	.4349043	0.875	0.381	.7015639	2.525297
sex	.859666	.266682	C	0.626	F	G

Stratified by ps

Model 2

Iteration 0: log likelihood = −188.55165

Stratified Cox regr. -- Breslow method for ties

No. of subjects =	76	Number of obs	=	76
No. of failures =	63			
Time at risk =	32380			
		LR chi2(7)	=	11.72
Log likelihood = −182.68981		Prob > chi2	=	0.1100

_t _d	Haz. Ratio	Std. Err.	z	P>|z|	[95% Conf. Interval]	
age	.997813	.0130114	−0.168	0.867	.9726342	1.023644
wtchg	.9322795	.329234	−0.199	0.843	.4666001	1.86272
sex	.782026	.2646556	−0.727	0.468	.4028608	1.518055
Ihist_2	.7627185	.4007818	−0.515	0.606	.2723251	2.136195
Ihist_3	4.168391	2.87634	2.069	0.039	1.077975	16.11863
Ihist_4	.9230807	.5042144	−0.147	0.884	.3164374	2.692722
Ihist_5	5.550076	5.264405	1.807	0.071	.8647887	35.6195

Stratified by ps

1. What is likelihood ratio chi-square for histologic type, with its degrees of freedom?
2. What is the hazard ratio of dying for patients with Histology type 2, compared to Histology type 1, with a confidence interval?
3. What is the change in risk of dying for an individual relative to someone 10 years younger?

References

1 Swinscow TDV. *Statistics at Square One, 9th edn* (revised by MJ Campbell). London: BMJ Books, 1996.
2 Collett D. *Modelling Survival Data in Medical Research.* London: Chapman and Hall, 1994.
3 Parmar MK, Machin D. *Survival Analysis: a practical approach.* Chichester: John Wiley, 1995.
4 Cox DR. Regression models and life tables (with discussion). *J Roy Statist Soc B* 1972; **34**: 187–220.

5   McIllmurray MB, Turkie E. Controlled trial of γ-linolenic acid in Dukes' C colorectal cancer. *BMJ* 1987; **294**: 1260; **295**: 475.
6   Oddy WH, Holt PG, Sly PD, Read AW, Landau LI, Stanley FJ, Kendall GE, Burton PR. Association between breast feeding and asthma in 6 year old children: findings of a prospective birth cohort study. *BMJ* 1999; **319**: 815–19.
7   STATACorp. STATA Statistical Software release 6.0. College Station, TX: Stata Corporation, 1999.
8   Piantadosi A. *Clinical Trials: a methodologic perspective.* Chichester: John Wiley, 1997.

5 Random effects models

Summary

Random effects models are useful in the analysis of repeated measures studies and cluster randomised trials, where the observations can be grouped, and within the group they are not independent. Ignoring the clustering can lead to underestimation of the standard error of key estimates. There are two types of models: *cluster-specific* and *marginal models*. Marginal models are easier to fit and utilise a technique known as *generalised estimating equations (gee)*.

5.1 Introduction

The models described so far only have one error term. In multiple regression, as described by model (2.1) the error term was an explicit variable, ε, added to the predictor. In logistic regression, the error was Binomial and described how the observed and predicted values were related. However it is possible for there to be more than one error term. A simple example of this is when observations are repeated over time on individuals. There is then the random variation *within individuals* (repeating an observation on an individual does not necessarily give the same answer) and random variation *due to individuals* (one individual differs from another). Another example would be where doctors each treat a number of patients. There is *within-doctor variation* (since patients vary) and *between-doctor variation* (since different doctors are likely to have different effects). These are often known as *hierarchical data structures* since there is a natural hierarchy, with one set of observations nested within another. One form of model used to fit data of this kind is known as a *random effects model*. In recent years there has been a great deal of interest in this type of model, and results are now regularly appearing in the medical literature. This chapter can no more than alert the reader to the importance of the topic.

5.2 Models for random effects

Consider a randomised trial, where there are single measurements on individuals, but the individuals form distinct groups, such as being treated by a particular doctor. For continuous outcomes y_{ij} for an individual j in group i we assume that

$$y_{ij} = \beta_0 + z_i + \beta_1 x_{1ij} + \ldots + \beta_p x_{pij} + \varepsilon_{ij} \tag{5.1}$$

This model is very similar to equation 2.1, with the addition of an extra term z_i.

Here z_i is assumed to be a random variable with $E(z_i) = 0$, $\text{Var}(z_i) = \sigma_B^2$ and reflects the overall effect of being in group i, where B indicates Between groups. The x_{kij}s are the covariates on the kth covariate on the jth individual in the ith group with regression coefficients β_k.

We assume

$$\text{Var}(\varepsilon_{ij}) = \sigma^2 \text{ and thus Var }(y_{ij}) = \sigma^2 + \sigma_B^2$$

Thus the variability of an observation has two components, the within and between group variances.

The observations within a group are correlated and

$$\text{Corr}(y_{ij} y_{ik}) = \rho = \frac{\sigma_B^2}{\sigma^2 + \sigma_B^2} \text{ if } j \text{ and } k \text{ differ}$$

This is known as the *intra-cluster (group) correlation (ICC)*.

It can be shown that when a model is fitted which ignores each z_i the standard error of the estimate of β_i is usually too small, and thus in general is likely to increase the Type I error rate. In particular, if all the groups are of the same size, m, then the variance of the estimate increases by $(1 + (m-1)\rho)$ and this is known as the *design effect (DE)*.

For some methods of fitting the model we need to assume also that z_i and ε_{ij} are Normally distributed, but this is not always the case.

Model (5.1) is often known as the *random intercepts model*, since the intercepts are $\beta_0 + z_i$ for different groups i and these vary randomly. They are a subgroup of what is known as *multi-level models*, since the different error terms can be thought of as being different levels of a hierarchy, individuals nested within groups. They are also called *mixed models* because they mix random effects and fixed effects. Model (5.1) is called an *exchangeable model* because it would not affect the estimation procedure if two observations within a cluster were exchanged. Another way of looking at exchangeability, is that from equation (5.1), given a value for z_i, the correlation between y_{ij} and $y_{ij'}$ is the same for any individuals j and j' in the same group.

Another type of model is known as a *random coefficient model*, where we assume that a slope, say β_1 can be described as a random variable, rather than a fixed population value. These are beyond the scope of this book.

Further details of these models are given in Brown and Prescott.[1] Repeated measures are described in Crowder and Hand,[2] and Diggle, Liang and Zeger.[3] Hierarchical models are described by Goldstein.[4]

5.3 Random vs fixed effects

Suppose we wish to include a variable in a model that covers differing groups of individuals. It could be a generic description, such as "smokers" or "non-smokers" or it could be quite specific, such as patients treated by Doctor A or Doctor B. The conventional method of allowing for categorical variables is to fit dummy variables as described in Chapter 2. This is known as a *fixed-effect model*, because the effect of being in a particular group is assumed fixed, and represented by a fixed population parameter. Thus "smoking" will decrease lung function by a certain amount on average. Being cared for by Doctor A may also affect your lung function, particularly if you are asthmatic. However, Doctor A's effect is of no interest to the world at large, in fact is only so much extra noise in the study. However, the effect of smoking is of interest generally. The main difference between a fixed and a random effect model depends on the intention of the analysis. If the study were repeated, would the same groups be used again? If not, then a random effect model is appropriate. By fitting dummy variables we are removing the effect of the differing groups as confounders but if these groups are unique to this study, and in a new study there will be a different set of groups, then we are pretending accuracy that we do not have. Thus random effects are sources of "error" in a model due to individuals or groups over and above the unit "error" term.

5.4 Use of random effects models

5.4.1 Cluster randomised trials

A cluster randomised trial is one in which groups of patients are randomised to an intervention or control, rather than individual patients. The group may be a geographical area, a general or family practice or a school. A general practice trial actively involves general practitioners and their primary healthcare teams, and the unit of randomisation may be the practice or healthcare professional rather than the patient. The effectiveness of the intervention is assessed in terms of the outcome for the patient.

There are many different features associated with cluster randomised trials and some of the statistical aspects were first discussed by Cornfield.[5] A useful discussion has been given by Zucker et al.[6] The main feature is that patients treated by one healthcare professional tend to be more similar than those treated by different healthcare professionals. If we know which doctor a patient is being treated by we can predict slightly better than by chance the performance of the patient and thus the observations for one doctor are not completely independent. What is surprising is how even a small correlation can greatly affect the design and analysis of such studies. For example with an ICC of 0.05 (a value commonly found in general practice trials), and 20 patients per group, the usual standard error estimate for a treatment effect, ignoring the effect of clustering, will be about 30% lower than a valid estimate should be. This greatly increases the chance of getting a significant result even when there is no real effect (a Type I error).

Further discussion on the uses and problems of cluster randomised trials in general (family) practice has been given recently.[7]

5.4.2 Repeated measures

A repeated measures study is where the same variable is observed on more than one occasion on each individual. An example might be a clinical trial to reduce blood pressure, where the blood pressure is measured 3, 6, 12 and 24 weeks after treatment. Each individual will have an effect on blood pressure, measured by the variable z_i. The individuals themselves are a sample from a population, and the level of blood pressure of a particular individual is not of interest.

A simple method of analysing data of this type is by means of summary measures.[8,9] Using this method we simply find a summary measure for each individual, often just the average, and analyse this as the primary outcome variable. This then eliminates the within individual variability, and so we have only one error term, due to between individual variation, to consider. Other summary values might be the maximum value attained over the time period, or the slope of the line. For repeated measures the data are collected in order, and the order may be important. Model (5.1) can be extended to allow for so-called *autoregressive models* which take account of the ordering, but that is beyond the scope of this book.

5.4.3 Sample surveys

Another simple use of the models would be in a sample survey, for example to find out levels of depression in primary care. A random sample of practices is chosen and within them a random sample of patients. The effect of being cared for by a particular practice on an individual is not of prime interest. If we repeated the study we would have a different set of practices. However, the variation induced on the estimate of the proportion of depressed patients by different practices *is* of interest, because it will affect the confidence interval. Thus we need to allow for between practice variation in our overall estimate.

5.5 Random effects models in action

5.5.1 Cluster trials

Diabetes from diagnosis was a study of patient centred intervention for the treatment of newly diagnosed diabetics.[10] Briefly, 41 practices were recruited and randomised into two groups: 21 in the intervention and 20 in the comparison arm. In the intervention group the health professionals were given 1.5 days' group training introducing the evidence for and skills of patient-centred care. They were also give a patient-held booklet which encouraged asking questions. The other group were simply given the British Diabetic Association guidelines on the management of newly diagnosed diabetics. There were a number of outcomes such as the HbA1c, the body mass index (BMI) at one year after intervention and process measures such as patient satisfaction. The important points are that patients treated by a particular doctor will tend to have more similar outcomes than patients treated by different doctors, and the trial is of an intervention package that would be given to different doctors in any future implementation. The effect of the intervention was a difference in BMI at one year of $1.90 \, \text{kg/m}^2$ in the two groups (SE 0.82). With no allowance for clustering the standard error was 0.76, which magnifies the apparent significance of the effect.

5.5.2 Repeated measures

Doull et al.[11] looked at the growth rate of 50 children with asthma before and after taking inhaled steroids. They showed that, compared to before treatment, the difference in growth rate between weeks 0 to 6 after treatment was -0.067 mm/week (95% CI -0.12 to -0.015), whereas at weeks 19 to 24, compared to before treatment it was -0.002 (95% CI -0.054 to 0.051). This showed that the growth suppressive action of inhaled corticosteroids is relatively short lived. The random effect model enabled a random child effect to be included in the model. It allowed differing numbers of measurements per child to be accounted for. The model gives increased confidence that the results can be generalised beyond these particular children.

5.6 Ordinary least squares at the group level

Cornfield[5] stated that one should "analyse as you randomise". Since randomisation is at the level of the group, a simple analysis would be to calculate "summary measures" such as the mean value for each group, and analyse these as the primary outcome variable.

Omitting the covariates from the model for simplicity, except for a dummy variable δ_i which takes the value 1 for the intervention and 0 for the control, it can be shown that

$$\bar{y}_i = \mu + \tau\delta_i + \bar{\varepsilon}_i \tag{5.2}$$

where $\bar{y}_i$ is the mean value for the n_i individuals with outcome y_{ij} for group i and

$$\text{Var}(\bar{y}_i) = \sigma_B^2 + \frac{\sigma^2}{n_i}$$

Equation (5.2) is a simple model with independent errors, which are homogeneous if each n_i is of similar size. An ordinary least squares estimate at group level of τ is unbiased and the standard error of estimate is valid provided the error term is independent of the treatment effect.

Thus, a simple analysis at the group level would be the following: if each n_i the same or not too different carries out a two sample t test on the group level means. This is the method of summary measures mentioned in section 5.4.2. It is worth noting that if σ^2 is zero (all values from a group are the same) then group size does not matter.

There are a number of problems with a group level approach. The main one is, how should individual level covariates be allowed for? It is unsatisfactory to use group averaged values of the individual level covariates. This method ignores the fact that the summary measures may be estimated with different precision for different individuals. The advantage of random effects models over summary measures is that they can allow for covariates which may vary with individuals. They also allow for different numbers of individuals per group.

5.7 Computer analysis

5.7.1 Likelihood and generalised estimating equations

Many computer packages will now fit random effects models although different packages may use different methods of fitting model (5.1). The likelihood method first assumes a distribution (usually Normal) for each z_i and then formulates a probability of observing each y_{ij} conditional on each z_i. Using the distribution of each z_i we can obtain an expected probability over every possible z_i. This involves mathematical integration and is difficult. Since the method calculates the regression coefficients separately for each group or cluster, this is often known as the *cluster-specific model*. A simpler method is known as *generalised estimating equations (gee)* which does not require Normality of the random effects. This method essentially uses the mean values per group as the outcome, and adjusts the standard error for the comparison to allow for within group correlation using what is known as a *robust sandwich estimator*. The gee methodology is based on what is known as a *marginal model*. In an ordinary table of data, the edges of the table are the margins and they contain the mean values; hence the name marginal model. The gee methodology uses the means per group, with the correlations within a group as a nuisance factor. Because the group is the main item for analysis, gee methodology may be unreliable unless the number of clusters exceeds 20, and preferably 40.

The methods can be extended to allow for binomial errors, so that one can get random effect logistic regression. The maximum likelihood method is less likely to be available in computer packages for logistic regression, and most packages at present only offer gee methods.

Murray[12] gives extensive programs using the computer package SAS for fitting the random effects models. STATA[13] devotes a whole suite of programs to what it calls *cross-sectional time-series models*, but are essentially repeated measures or clustered data. This type of model is generalised quite naturally to a Bayesian approach (see Appendix 4). This is beyond the scope of this book but further details are given in Turner, Omar and Thompson.[14]

5.7.2 Interpreting computer output

Table 5.1 gives some data which are a subset of data from Kinmonth *et al.*[10] They consist of the body mass index at one year on a number of patients in 10 practices, under one of two treatment groups.

The results are shown in Table 5.2. Table 5.2(i) shows the results of fitting an ordinary regression without clustering, which yields an estimate of a treatment effect of 0.42, with standard error 1.90. As was stated earlier, since this ignores the clustering inherent in the data the standard error will be too small. Table 5.2(ii) shows the

Table 5.1 Data on body mass index.[10]

Subject	BMI (kg/m^2)	Treatment	Practice
1	26.2	1	1
2	27.1	1	1
3	25.0	1	2
4	28.3	1	2
5	30.5	1	3
6	28.8	1	4
7	31.0	1	4
8	32.1	1	4
9	28.2	1	5
10	30.9	1	5
11	37.0	0	6
12	38.1	0	6
13	22.1	0	7
14	23.0	0	7
15	23.2	0	8
16	25.7	0	8
17	27.8	0	9
18	28.0	0	9
19	28.0	0	10
20	31.0	0	10

results of fitting a maximum likelihood model, which yields an estimate of the treatment effect of 0.39, with standard error 2.47. Note how the standard error is greatly inflated compared to the model that fails to allow for clustering. The program also gives an estimate of the intra-cluster correlation coefficient, rho, of 0.85 and the between and within groups standard deviations, here denoted sigma_u and sigma_e. The output also states the random effects are assumed Gaussian, which is a synonym for Normal (after C.F. Gauss, a German mathematician who first described the distribution). Using the method of generalised estimating equations in Table 5.2(iii) also yields a treatment estimate of 0.39, but a standard error of 2.61. As described earlier, the assumption underlying this model is that individuals within a group are *exchangeable*. The estimate from gee can be contrasted with the method which uses the average per group as the outcome in Table 5.2(iv). This yields an estimate of 0.41, with an even larger standard error of 2.74.

Table 5.2 Computer output fitting regression models to data in Table 5.1.

(i) Regression not allowing for clustering

Source	SS	df	MS		
Model	.881999519	1	.881999519		
Residual	326.397937	18	18.1332187		
Total	327.279937	19	17.2252598		

Number of obs = 20
F(1, 18) = 0.05
Prob > F = 0.8279
R-squared = 0.0027
Adj R-squared = -0.0527
Root MSE = 4.2583

bmi	Coef.	Std. Err.	t	P>|t|	[95% Conf. Interval]
treat	.4199999	1.904375	0.221	0.828	-3.580943 4.420943
_cons	28.39	1.346596	21.083	0.000	25.56091 31.21909

(ii) Maximum likelihood random effects model

Fitting constant-only model:
Iteration 0:   log likelihood = −51.281055
Iteration 4:   log likelihood = −49.644194

Fitting full model:
Iteration 0:   log likelihood = −51.269825
Iteration 4:   log likelihood = −49.631613

Random-effects ML regression   Number of obs   =   20
Group variable (i) : group   Number of groups   =   10

Random effects u_i ~ Gaussian   Obs per group: min   =   1
                                                      avg   =   2.0
                                                      max   =   3
                                      LR chi2(1)   =   0.03
Log likelihood = −49.631613   Prob > chi2   =   0.8740

bmi	Coef.	Std. Err.	z	P>|z|	[95% Conf. Interval]
treat	.3916501	2.467672	0.159	0.874	-4.444899 5.228199
_cons	28.39	1.740882	16.308	0.000	24.97793 31.80207
/sigma_u	3.737395	.9099706	4.107	0.000	1.953885 5.520904
/sigma_e	1.539626	.3430004	4.489	0.000	.8673579 2.211895
rho	.854917	.0848639			.6286473 .9630508

Likelihood ratio test of sigma_u=0: chi2(1) = 13.34 Prob > chi2 = 0.0003

(iii) generalised estimating equations

Iteration 1: tolerance = .01850836
Iteration 2: tolerance = .0000438
Iteration 3: tolerance = 1.029e-07

GEE population-averaged model			Number of obs	=	20
Group variable:	group		Number of groups	=	10
Link:	identity		Obs per group: min	=	1
Family:	Gaussian		avg	=	2.0
Correlation:	exchangeable		max	=	3
			Wald chi2(1)	=	0.02
Scale parameter:	18.1336		Prob > chi2	=	0.8803

bmi	Coef.	Std. Err.	z	P>|z|	[95% Conf. Interval]	
treat	.3937789	2.613977	0.151	0.880	−4.729523	5.51708
_cons	28.39	1.844712	15.390	0.000	24.77443	32.00557

(iv) Regression on group means
Between regression

(regression on group means)		Number of obs	=	20
Group variable (i) : group		Number of groups	=	10

R-sq: within =	.	Obs per group: min	=	1
between =	0.0027	avg	=	2.0
overall =	0.0027	max	=	3
		F(1,8)	=	0.02
sd(u_i + avg(e_i.)) =	4.34548	Prob > F	=	0.8860

bmi	Coef.	Std. Err.	t	P>|t|	[95% Conf. Interval]	
treat	.4066669	2.748323	0.148	0.886	−5.930976	6.74431
_cons	28.39	1.943358	14.609	0.000	23.90861	32.87139

The methods will give increasingly different results as the variation between groups increases. In this example the estimate of the treatment effect is quite similar for each method, but the standard errors vary somewhat.

5.8 Model checking

Most of the assumptions for random effects models are similar to those of linear or logistic models described in Chapters 2 and 3.

The main difference is in the assumptions underlying the random term. Proper checking is beyond the scope of this book, but the maximum likelihood method assumes that the random terms are distributed Normally. If the numbers of measurements per cluster are fairly uniform, then a simple check would be to examine the cluster means, in a histogram. This is difficult to interpret if the numbers per cluster vary a great deal. In cluster randomised trials, it would be useful to check that the numbers of patients per cluster are not affected by treatment. Sometimes, when the intervention is a training package, for example, the effect of training is to increase recruitment to the trial, so leading to an imbalance in the treatment and control arms.

5.9 Reporting the results of a random effects analysis

- Give the number of *groups* as well as the number of individuals.

- In a cluster randomised trial, give the group level means of covariates by treatment arm, so the reader can see if the trial is balanced *at a group level*.

- Describe whether a cluster specific or a marginal model is being used and justify the choice.

- Indicate how the assumptions underlying the distribution of the random effects were verified.

5.10 Reading about the results of a random effects analysis

- What is the main unit of analysis? Does the statistical analysis reflect this? Repeating a measurement on one individual is not the same as making the second measurement on a different individual, and the statistical analysis should be different in each situation.

- If the study is a cluster randomised trial, was an appropriate model used?

- If the analysis uses gee methodology, are there sufficient groups to justify the results?

Frequently asked question

When should I use a random effects model?

There is currently still much debate on the use of random effects models. In repeated measures data and cluster randomised trials they would seem to be the models of choice. However, there are other areas where their use is still controversial. For example, the pooling of the results from four studies described in Table 3.3, is an example of *meta-analysis*. The four studies could be regarded as four samples from a larger pool of potential case–control studies, and so a random effects model may seem appropriate. However, this is not universally accepted, and it is wise to consult an experienced statistician for advice on these issues.

References

1 Brown H, Prescott R. *Applied Mixed Models in Medicine*. Chichester: John Wiley, 1999.
2 Crowder M, Hand DJ. *Analysis of Repeated Measures*. London: Chapman and Hall, 1999.
3 Diggle PJ, Liang K-Y, Zeger S. *Analysis of Longitudinal Data*. Oxford: Oxford Science Publications, 1994.
4 Goldstein H. *Multi-level Models, 2nd edn*. London: Arnold, 1996.
5 Cornfield J. Randomization by group: a formal analysis. *Am J Epidemiol* 1978; **108**: 100–2.
6 Zucker DM, Lakatos E, Webber LS *et al*. Statistical Design of the Child and Adolescent Trial for Cardiovascular Health (CATCH): implications of cluster randomization. *Control Clin Trials* 1995; **16**: 96–118.
7 Campbell MJ. Cluster randomised trials in general (family) practice. *Stat Methods Med Res* 2000; **9**: 81–94.
8 Matthews JNS, Altman DG, Campbell MJ, Royston JP. Analysis of serial measurements in medical research. *BMJ* 1990; **300:** 230–5.
9 Campbell MJ, Machin D. *Medical Statistics: a commonsense approach, 3rd edn*. Chichester: John Wiley, 1999.

10 Kinmonth AL, Woodcock A, Griffin S, Spiegal N, Campbell MJ. Randomised controlled trial of patient centred care of diabetes in general practice: impact on current wellbeing and future disease risk. *BMJ* 1998; **317**: 1202–8.

11 Doull IJM, Campbell MJ, Holgate ST. Duration of growth suppressive effects of regular inhaled corticosteroids *Arch Dis Child* 1998; **78**: 172–3.

12 Murray DM. *Design and Analysis of Community Trials.* Oxford: Oxford University Press, 1998.

13 STATACorp. STATA Statistical Software. 6.0 1999 Reference Manual. College Station, TX: STATA Corporation 1999, Section 23.11.

14 Turner RM, Omar RZ, Thompson SG. Bayesian methods of analysis for cluster randomised trials with binary outcome data. *Statistics in Medicine* (in press), 2001.

6 Other models

Summary

This chapter will consider three other regression models that are of considerable use in medical research: *Poisson regression, ordinal regression* and *time-series regression*. Poisson regression is useful when the outcome variable is a count. Ordinal regression is useful when the outcome is ordinal, or ordered categorical. Time-series regression is mainly used when the outcome is continuous, but measured together with the predictor variables serially over time.

6.1 Poisson regression

Poisson regression is an extension of logistic regression where the risk of an event to an individual is small, but there are a large number of individuals, so the number of events in a group is appreciable. We need to know not just whether an individual had an event, but for how long they were followed up, the *person-years*. This is sometimes known as the amount of time they were *at risk*. It is used extensively in epidemiology, particularly in the analysis of cohort studies. For further details see McNeil.[1]

6.1.1 The model

The outcome for a Poisson model is a count of events in a group, usually over a period of time, for example number of deaths over 20 years in a group exposed to asbestos. It is a *discrete quantitative variable* in the terminology of Chapter 1. The principal covariate is a measure of the amount of time the group has been in the study. Subjects may have been in the study for differing lengths of time (known as the *at risk period*) and so we record the time each individual is observed to give an exposure time e_i. In logistic regression we modelled the probability of an event π_i. Here we model the underlying rate λ_i which is the number of events expected to occur E_i over a period i divided by the time e_i. Instead of a logistic transform we use a simple log transform.

The model is

$$\log(\lambda_i) = \log(E_i/e_i) = \beta_0 + \beta_1 X_{i1} + \ldots + \beta_p X_{ip} \qquad (6.1)$$

This may be rewritten as

$$E_i = \exp\{\log(e_i) + \beta_0 + \beta_1 X_{i1} + \ldots + \beta_p X_{ip}\} \qquad (6.2)$$

It is assumed that risk of an event rises directly with e_i and so in the model (6.2) the coefficient for $\log(e_i)$ is fixed at 1. This is known as an *offset* and is a special type of independent variable whose regression coefficient is fixed at unity.

Note that, as for the logistic regression, the *observed counts* have not yet appeared in the model. They are linked to the expected counts by the Poisson distribution (see Appendix 2). Thus we assume that the observed count y_i is distributed as a Poisson variable with parameter $E_i = \lambda_i e_i$.

Instead of a measure of the person-years at risk, we could use the predicted number of deaths, based on external data. For example we could use the age/sex specific death rates for England & Wales to predict the number of deaths in each group. This would enable us to model the *standardised mortality ratio (SMR)*. For further details see Breslow and Day.[2]

6.1.2 Consequences of the model

Consider a cohort study in which the independent variable is a simple binary 0 or 1, respectively, for people not exposed or exposed to a hazard. The dependent variable is whether they succumb to disease and we also have the length of time they were on study. Then the coefficient b estimated from the model is the log of the ratio of the estimated incidence of the disease in those exposed and not exposed. Thus $\exp(b)$ is the estimated *incidence rate ratio (irr)* or *relative risk*. If the independent variable is continuous then the regression coefficient measures the *percentage change* of the y variable per unit increase of the independent variable.

6.1.3 Interpreting a computer output

The data layout is exactly the same as for the grouped logistic regression described in Chapter 3. The model is fitted by maximum likelihood.

Table 6.1 gives data from the classic cohort study of coronary deaths and smoking amongst British male doctors,[3] quoted in Breslow and Day[2] and McNeil.[1]

Table 6.1 Coronary deaths from British male doctors.

Deaths (D)	Person-years	Smoker	Age-group at start study	Expected (E)	$(D-E) \div \sqrt{E}$
32	52407	1	35–44	27.2	0.92
2	18790	0	35–44	6.8	−1.85
104	43248	1	45–54	98.9	0.52
12	10673	0	45–54	17.1	−1.24
206	28612	1	55–64	205.3	0.05
28	5712	0	55–64	28.7	−0.14
186	12663	1	65–74	187.2	−0.09
28	2585	0	65–74	26.8	0.23
102	5317	1	75–84	111.5	−0.89
31	1462	0	75–84	21.5	2.05

Here the question is what is the risk of deaths associated with smoking, allowing for age? Thus the dependent variable is number of deaths per age/smoking group. Smoking group is the causal variable, age group is a confounder and the person-years is the offset. The analysis is given in Table 6.2.

The five age groups have been fitted using four dummy variables, with age group 35–44 years as the baseline. The model used here assumes that the relative risk of coronary death for smokers remains constant for each age group. The estimated relative risk for smokers compared to non-smokers is 1.43, with 95% confidence interval 1.16 to 1.76 which is highly significant (P=0.001). Thus male British doctors are 40% more likely to die of a coronary death if they smoke. The LR chi-squared is an overall test of the model and is highly significant, but this significance is largely due to the age categories — coronary risk is highly age dependent. It has five parameters because there are five parameters in this particular model. Note, the output is similar to that for survival analysis, and the z statistic is *not* the ratio of the IRR to its standard error, but rather the ratio of the log(IRR), (log(1.43)) to *its* standard error.

Table 6.2 Results of Poisson regression on data in Table 6.1.

Iteration 0:	log likelihood	=	−33.823578
Iteration 1:	log likelihood	=	−33.60073
Iteration 2:	log likelihood	=	−33.600412
Iteration 3:	log likelihood	=	−33.600412

Poisson regression

				Number of obs	=	10
				LR chi2(5)	=	922.93
				Prob > chi2	=	0.0000
Log likelihood = −33.600412				Pseudo R2	=	0.9321

y	IRR	Std. Err.	z	P>|z|	[95% Conf.	Interval]
smoker	1.425664	.1530791	3.303	0.001	1.155102	1.7596
Age 45-54	4.41056	.860515	7.606	0.000	3.008995	6.464962
Age 55-64	13.83849	2.542506	14.301	0.000	9.65384	19.83707
Age 65-74	28.51656	5.269837	18.130	0.000	19.85162	40.96364
Age 75-84	40.45104	7.77548	19.249	0.000	27.75314	58.95862
pyrs	(exposure)					

6.1.4 Model checking

The simplest way to check the model is to compare the observed values and those predicted by the model. The predicted values are obtained by putting the estimated coefficients into equation (6.2). Since the dependent variable is a count we can use a chi-squared test to compare the observed and predicted values and we obtain $X^2 = 12.13$, df=4, P=0.0164. This has 4 degrees of freedom because the predicted values are constrained to equal the observed values for the five age groups and one smoking group (the other smoking group constraint follows from the previous age group constraints). Thus six constraints and ten observations yield 4 degrees of freedom. There is some evidence that the model does not fit the data. The standardised residuals are defined as $(D-E)/\sqrt{E}$ since the standard error of D is $\sqrt{E}$. These are shown in Table 6.1 and we expect most to lie between -2 and $+2$. We can conclude there is little evidence of a systematic lack of fit of the model, except possibly for the non-smokers in the age group 75–84 years, but this is not a large difference.

The only additional term we have available to fit is the smoking $\times$ age interaction. This yields a saturated model (i.e. one in which the number of parameters equals the number of data points, see Appendix 2), and its LR chi-squared is equal to the lack of fit chi-squared above. Thus there is some evidence that smoking affects coronary risk differently at different ages.

When the observed data vary from the predicted values by more than would be expected by a Poisson distribution we have what is known as *extra-Poisson variation*. This is similar to *extra-Binomial variation* described in Chapter 3. It means that the standard errors given by the computer output may not be valid. It may arise because an important covariate is omitted. Another common explanation is when the counts are correlated. This can happen when they refer to counts *within* an individual, such as number of asthma attacks per year, rather than counts within groups of separate individuals. This leads to a random effects model as described in Chapter 5 which, as explained there, will tend to increase our estimate of the standard error. Some packages now allow one to fit random effect Poisson models. A particular model that allows for extra variation in λ_i is known as *negative Binomial regression* and this is available in STATA, for example.

6.1.5 Poisson regression in action

Campbell *et al.*[4] looked at deaths from asthma over the period 1980–1995 in England & Wales. They used Poisson regression to test whether there was a trend in the deaths over the period, and concluded that, particularly for the age group 15–44, there had been a decline of about 6% (95% CI 5% to 7%) per year since 1988, but this downward trend was not evident in the elderly.

6.2 Ordinal regression

When the outcome variable is *ordinal* then the methods described in the earlier chapters are inadequate. One solution would be to dichotomise the data and use logistic regression as discussed in Chapter 3. However, this is inefficient and possibly biased if the point for the dichotomy is chosen by looking at the data. The main model for ordinal regression is known as the *proportional odds* or *cumulative logit model*. It is based on the cumulative response probabilities rather than the category probabilities.

For example, consider an ordinal outcome variable Y with k ordered categorical outcomes y_j denoted by $j=1,2,...,k$, and let $X_1,...X_p$ denote the covariates. The cumulative logit or proportional odds model is

$$\text{logit}(C_j)=\log\left[\frac{C_j}{1-C_j}\right]=\log\left[\frac{Pr(Y\leq y_j)}{Pr(Y.y_j)}\right]=\alpha_j+\beta_1X_1+...+\beta_pX_p,$$

$$(6.3) \quad j=1,2,...,k-1$$

or equivalently as

$$Pr(Y\leq y_j)=\frac{\exp(\alpha_j+\beta_1X_1+...+\beta_pX_p)}{1+\exp(\alpha_j+\beta_1X_1+...+\beta_pX_p)} \quad j=1,2,...,k-1 \qquad (6.4)$$

where $C_j=Pr(Y\leq y_j)$ is the cumulative probability of being in category j or less (note that for $j=k$; $Pr(Y\leq y_j|X)=1$). Here we have not used coefficients to indicate individuals to avoid cluttering the notation. Note we have replaced the intercept term β_0 which would be seen in logistic regression by a set of variables $\alpha_j, j=1,2,...k-1$. When there are $k=2$ categories, this model is identical to equation (3.1), the logistic regression model. When there are more than two categories, we estimate separate intercepts terms for each category except the base category.

The regression coefficient vector β does not depend on the category i. This implies that the model (6.3) assumes that the relationship between the covariates x and Y is independent of i (the response category). This assumption of identical log-odds ratios across the k categories is known as the *proportional odds assumption*.

The proportional odds model is useful when one believes the dependent variable is continuous, but the values have been grouped for reporting. Alternatively the variable is measured imperfectly by an instrument with a limited number of values. The divisions between the boundaries are sometimes known as *cut-points*. The proportional odds model is invariant when the codes for the response Y are reversed (i.e. y_1 recoded as y_k, y_2 recoded as y_{k-1} and so on). Secondly the proportional odds model is invariant under the collapsibility of adjacent categories of the ordinal response (for example y_1 and y_2 combined and y_{k-1} and y_k combined).

Note that count data, described under Poisson regression, could be thought of as ordinal. However, ordinal regression is likely to be inefficient in this case because count data form a ratio scale, and this fact is not utilised in ordinal regression (see section 1.3).

The interpretation of the model is exactly like that of logistic regression. Continuous and nominal covariates can be included as independent variables.

6.2.1 Interpreting a computer output

Suppose the length of breast feeding given in Table 3.1 was measured as less than 1 month, 1–3 months and greater than or equal to 3 months. Thus the cut-points are 1 month and 3 months. The data are given in Table 6.3.

Table 6.3 Numbers of wives of printers and farmers who breast fed their babies for less than 1 month, 1-3 months or for 3 months or more.

Wife	< 1 month	1–3 months	≥ 3 months	Total
Printers' wives	20	16	14	50
Farmers' wives	15	15	25	55
Total	35	31	39	105

The outcome variable is now *ordinal* and it would be sensible to use an analysis that reflected this. In Swinscow,[5] we showed how this could be done using a non-parametric Mann–Whitney U test. Ordinal regression is equivalent to the Mann–Whitney test when there is only one independent variable 0/1 in the regression. The advantage of ordinal regression over non-parametric methods is that we get an efficient estimate of a regression coefficient and we can extend the analysis to allow for other confounding variables.

Table 6.4 Results of ordinal regression on data in Table 6.3.

```
Iteration 0:   log likelihood  =  −114.89615
Iteration 1:   log likelihood  =  −113.17681
Iteration 2:   log likelihood  =  −113.17539
```

Ordered logit estimates				Number of obs	=	105
				LR chi2(1)	=	3.44
				Prob > chi2	=	0.0636
Log likelihood= −113.17539				Pseudo R2	=	0.0150

breast	Coef.	Std. Err.	z	P>|z|	[95% Conf.	Interval]
treat	−.671819	.3643271	−1.844	0.065	−1.385887	.0422491
_cut1	−1.03708	.282662	(Ancillary parameters)			
_cut2	.2156908	.2632804				

For the analysis we coded printers' wives as 1 and farmers' wives as 0. The dependent variable was coded 1,2,3 but in fact many packages will allow any positive whole numbers. The computer analysis is given in Table 6.4. Alas the computer output does not give the odds ratios and so we have to compute them ourselves. Thus the odds ratio is $\exp(-0.672)=0.51$ with 95% CI as $\exp(-1.386)$ to $\exp(0.042)$, which is 0.25 to 1.04. This contrasts with the odds ratio of 0.47 (95% CI 0.21 to 1.05) that we obtained in Table 3.2 when we had only two categories for the dependent variable. The interpretation is that after 1 month, and after 3 months, a printer's wife has half the odds of being in the same breast feeding category *or higher* as a farmer's wife.

The LR chi-squared has one degree of freedom, corresponding to the single term in the model. The P value associated with it, 0.0636, agrees closely with the Wald P value of 0.065. The two intercepts are labelled in the output _cut1 and _cut2. They are known as *ancillary parameters*, meaning that they are extra parameters introduced to fit the model, but not part of the inferential study. Thus no significance levels are attached to them.

Useful discussions of the proportional odds model and other models for ordinal data have been given by Armstrong and Sloan[7] and Ananth and Kleinbaum.[6] Other models include the *continuation ratio model*. Armstong and Sloan[7] conclude that the gain in efficiency using a proportional odds model as opposed to logistic regression is often not great. The strategy of dichotomising an ordinal variable and using logistic regression has much to recommend it in terms of simplicity and ease of interpretation, unless the coefficient of the main predictor variable is close to borderline significance.

6.2.2 Model checking

Tests are available for proportional odds but these tests lack power. Also the model is robust to mild departures from the assumption of proportional odds. A crude test would be to examine the odds ratios associated with each cut-point. If they are all greater than unity, or all less than unity, then a proportional odds model will suffice. From Table 6.3 we find the odds are:

$$<1 \text{ month versus} \geq 1 \text{ month}$$
$$\text{Odds ratio} = \frac{15 \times 30}{20 \times 40} = 0.56$$

$$<3 \text{ months vs} \geq 3 \text{ months}$$
$$\text{Odds ratio} = \frac{30 \times 14}{36 \times 25} = 0.47$$

These odds ratios are quite close to each other and we can see that the observed odds ratio of 0.51 from the proportional odds model is midway between the two. Thus we have no reason to reject the proportional odds model. Model testing is much more complicated when there is more than one input variable and some of them are continuous, and specialist help should be sought.

6.2.3 Ordinal regression in action

Hotopf et al.[8] looked at the relationship between chronic childhood abdominal pain as measured on three consecutive surveys at ages 7, 11 and 15 and adult psychiatric disorders at the age of 36, in a cohort of 3637 individuals. A seven-point index of psychiatric disorder (the "index of definition") was measured as an outcome variable. This is an ordinal scale. It was found that the binary predictor (causal) variable, pain on all three surveys, was associated with an odds ratio of 2.72 (95% CI 1.65 to 4.49) when potential confounders sex, father's social class, marital status at age 36 and educational status were included in the model. Thus the authors conclude that children with abdominal pain are more likely to present psychiatric problems in later life. The usual cut-off for the index of definition is 5, but use of the whole scale uses more information and so gives more precise estimates.

6.3 Time-series regression

Time-series regression is concerned with the situation in which the dependent and independent variables are measured over time. Usually there is only a single series with one dependent variable and a number of independent variables, unlike repeated measures when there may be several series of data.

The potential for confounding in time-series regression is very high – many variables either simply increase or decrease over time, and so will be correlated over time.[9] In addition many epidemiological variables are seasonal, and this variation would be present even if the factors were not causally related. It is important that seasonality and trends are properly accounted for. Simply because the outcome variable is seasonal, it is impossible to ascribe causality because of seasonality of the predictor variable. For example, sudden infant deaths are higher in winter than in summer, but this does not imply that temperature is a causal factor; there are many other factors that might affect the result such as reduced daylight, or presence of viruses. However, if an unexpectedly cold winter is associated with an increase in sudden infant deaths, or very cold days are consistently followed after a short time by rises in the daily sudden infant death rate, then causality may possibly be inferred.

Often when confounding factors are correctly accounted for, the serial correlation of the residuals disappears; they appear serially correlated because of the association with a time-dependent predictor variable, and so conditional on this variable the residuals are independent. This is particularly likely for mortality data, where, except in epidemics, the individual deaths are unrelated. Thus one can often use conventional regression methods followed by a check for the serial correlation of the residuals and need only proceed further if there is clear evidence of a lack of independence.

If the inclusion of known or potential confounders fails to remove the serial correlation of the residuals, then it is known that ordinary least squares do not provide valid estimates of the standard errors of the parameters.

6.3.1 The model

For a continuous outcome suppose the model is

$$y_t = \beta_0 + \beta_1 X_{t1} + \ldots + \beta_p X_{tp} + v_t, t = 1, \ldots, n \qquad (6.5)$$

The main difference from equation (2.1) is that we now index time t rather than individuals. It is important to distinguish time points because whereas two individuals with the same covariates are interchangeable, you cannot swap, say Saturday with Sunday and expect the same results! We denote the error term by v_t and we assume that $v_t = \varepsilon_t - \alpha v_{t-1}$ where the ε_t are assumed independent Normally distributed variables with mean zero and variance σ^2 and α is a constant between -1 and $+1$. The error term is known as an *autoregressive process (of order 1)*. This model implies that the data are correlated in time, known as *serial correlation*. The effect of ignoring serial correlation is to provide artificially low estimates of the standard error of the regression coefficients and thus to imply significance more often than the significance level would suggest, under the null hypothesis of no association.

6.3.2 Estimation using correlated residuals

Given the above model, and assuming α is known, we can use a method of generalised least squares known as the *Cochrane–Orcutt procedure*.[10]

For simplicity, assume one independent variable and write $y^*_t = y_t - \alpha y_{t-1}$ and $x^*_t = X_t - \alpha X_{t-1}$. We can then obtain an estimate of β using ordinary least squares on y^*_t and x^*_t. However, since α will not usually be known it can be estimated from the ordinary least squares residuals e_t by

$$\alpha = \sum_{t=2}^{n} e_t e_{t-1} \Big/ \sum_{t=2}^{n} e^2_{t-1}$$

This leads to an iterative procedure in which we can construct a new set of transformed variables and thus a new set of regression estimates and so on until convergence. The iterative Cochrane–Orcutt procedure can be interpreted as a stepwise algorithm for computing maximum likelihood estimators of α and β where the initial observation y_1 is regarded as fixed. If the residuals are assumed to be Normally distributed then full maximum likelihood methods are available, which estimate α and β simultaneously. This can be generalised to higher-order autoregressive models and fitted in a number of computer packages, in particular SAS. However caution is advised in using this method when the autocorrelations are high, and it is worth making the point that an autoregressive error model "should not be used as a nostrum for models that simply do not fit".

There are more modern methods which do not assume the first point is fixed, but if the data set is long (say >50 points) then the improvement is minimal. These models can be generalised to outcomes which are counts but this is beyond the scope of this book and for further details see Campbell.[12]

Table 6.5 Results of Cochrane–Orcutt regression on data in Table 2.1 assuming points all belong to one individual equally spaced over time.

```
Iteration 0:  rho  =  0.0000
Iteration 1:  rho  =  0.0432
Iteration 2:  rho  =  0.0462
Iteration 3:  rho  =  0.0463
Iteration 4:  rho  =  0.0463
Iteration 5:  rho  =  0.0463
```

Cochrane-Orcutt AR(1) regression iterated estimates

Source	SS	df	MS		
				Number of obs =	14
				F(1, 12) =	29.29
Model	4841.31415	1	4841.31415	Prob > F =	0.0002
Residual	1983.76032	12	165.31336	R-squared =	0.7093
				Adj R-squared =	0.6851
Total	6825.07447	13	525.005728	Root MSE =	12.857

Deadspce	Coef.	Std. Err.	t	P>|t|	[95% Conf. Interval]
Height	1.160173	.2143853	5.412	0.000	.6930675 1.627279
_cons	−102.1168	31.78251	−3.213	0.007	−171.3649 -32.86861
rho	.0463493				

Durbin-Watson statistic (original)   1.834073
Durbin-Watson statistic (transformed) 1.901575

6.3.3 Interpreting a computer output

Suppose that the data on deadspace and height in Table 2.1 in fact referred to one individual followed up over time. Then the regression of deadspace against height is given in Table 6.5 using Cochrane–Orcutt regression. This method loses the first observation, and so the regression coefficient is not strictly comparable with that in Figure 2.1. Note that the output gives the number of observations as 14, not 15. Note also that the standard error, 0.214 obtained here, is much larger than the 0.180 obtained when the points can all be assumed to be independent. The estimate of α, the autocorrelation coefficient is denoted rho in the printout and is quite small at 0.046. However the program does not give a P value for rho.

6.4 Reporting Poisson, ordinal or time-series regression in the literature

- If the dependent variable is discrete quantitative then Poisson regression may be the required model. Give evidence that the model is a reasonable fit to the data by quoting the goodness of fit chi-squared. Test for covariate interaction or allow for extra-Poisson variation if the model is not a good fit.

- If the dependent variable is ordinal, then ordinal regression *may* be useful. However if the ordinal variable has a large number of categories (say more than seven) then linear regression may be suitable. Give evidence that the proportional odds model is a reasonable one, perhaps by quoting the odds ratios associated with each cut-point for the main independent variable. If proportional odds is unlikely, then dichotomise the dependent variable and use logistic regression. *Do not* choose the point for dichotomy by choosing the one that gives the most significant value for the primary independent variable!

- When the data form a time series, look for evidence that the residuals in the model are serially correlated. If they are, then include a term in the model to allow for serial correlation.

6.5 Reading about the results of Poisson, ordinal or time-series regression in the literature

- As usual, look for evidence that the model is reasonable.

- In Poisson regression, are the counts independent? If not, should overdispersion be considered?

- If ordinal regression has been used, how has the result been interpreted?

- A common error in time series regression is to ignore serial correlation. This may not invalidate the analysis, but it is worth asking whether it might. Another common feature is to only use a first order autoregression to allow for serial correlation, but it may be worth asking whether this is sufficient.

References

1 McNeil D. *Epidemiological Research Methods*. Chichester: John Wiley, 1996.

2 Breslow NE, Day NE. *Statistical Methods in Cancer Research: Vol II – the design and analysis of cohort studies*. Lyon: IARC, 1987.

3 Doll R, Hill AB. Mortality of British doctors in relation to smoking: observations on coronary thrombosis. *Nat Cancer Inst Monog* 1996; **19**: 205–68.

4 Campbell MJ, Cogman GR, Holgate ST, Johnston SL. Age specific trends in asthma mortality in England & Wales 1983–1995: results of an observational study. *BMJ* 1997; **314**: 1439–41.

5 Swinscow TDV. *Statistics at Square One, 9th edn* (revised by MJ Campbell). London: BMJ Books, 1996.

6 Armstrong BG, Sloan M. Ordinal regression models for epidemiologic data. *Am J Epidemiol* 1989; **129**: 191–204.

7 Ananth CV, Kleinbaum DG. Regression models for ordinal responses: a review of methods and applications. *Int J Epidemiol* 1997; **26**: 1323–33.

8 Hotopf M, Carr S, Magou R, Wadsworth M, Wessely S. Why do children have chronic abdominal pain and what happens to them when they grow up? Population based cohort study. *BMJ* 1998; **316**: 1196–200.

9 Yule GU. Why do we sometimes get nonsense correlations between time series? A study in sampling and the nature of time-series. *J Roy Statist Soc* 1926; **89**: 187–227.

10 Cochrane D, Orcutt GH. Application of least squares regression to relationships containing autocorrelated error terms. *J Am Statist Assoc* 1949; **44**: 32–61.

11 SAS Institute Inc. *SAS/ETS User's Guide Version 5 Edition*. Cary, NC: SAS Institute, 1984: 192.

12 Campbell MJ. Time series regression. In: Armitage P, Cotton T, eds. *Encyclopaedia of Biostatistics*. Chichester: John Wiley, 1997: 4536–8.

Appendix 1
Exponentials and logarithms

Logarithms

It is simple to understand raising a quantity to a power, so that $y = x^2$ is equivalent to $y = x.x$. This can be generalised to $y = x^n$ for arbitrary n so $y^n = x.x... x$ n times.

A simple result is that

$$x^n.x^m = x^{n+m} \tag{A1.1}$$

for arbitrary n and m. Thus, for example $3^2 \times 3^4 = 3^6 = 729$. It can be shown that this holds for *any* values of m and n, not just whole numbers.

We define $x^0 = 1$, because $x^n = x^{0+n} = x^0 \, x^n = 1.x^n$.

A useful extension of the concept of powers is to let n take fractional or negative values. Thus $y = x^{0.5}$ can be shown to be equivalent to $y = \sqrt{x}$, because $x^{0.5}.x^{0.5} = x^{0.5+0.5} = x^1 = x$ and also $\sqrt{x}. \sqrt{x} = x$.

Also x^{-1} can be shown equivalent to $1/x$, because $x.x^{-1} = x^{1-1} = x^0 = 1$.

If $y = x^n$ then the definition of a logarithm of y to the base x is the power that x has to be raised to get y. This is written $n = \log_x(y)$ or "n equals log to the base x of y".

Suppose $y = x^n$ and $z = x^m$. It can be shown from equation (A1.1) that

$$\log_x(y.z) = n + m = \log_x(y) + \log_x(z)$$

Thus when multiplying two numbers we add their logs. This was the basis of the original use of logarithms in that they enabled a transformation whereby arithmetic using multiplications could be done using additions, which are much easier to do by hand. In Appendix 2 we need an equivalent result, namely that

103

$$\log_x(y/z) = \log_x(y) - \log_x(z)$$

In other words, when we log transform the ratio of two numbers we subtract the logs of the two numbers.

The two most common bases are 10, and a strange quantity $e = 2.718...$, where the dots indicate that the decimals go on indefinitely. This number has the useful property that the slope of the curve $y = e^x$ at any point (x, y) is just y, whereas for all other bases the slope is proportional to y but not exactly equal to it. The formula $y = e^x$ is often written $y = \exp(x)$. The logarithms to base e and 10 are often denoted ln and log on calculators, respectively, and the former is often called the *natural logarithm*. In this book all logarithms are natural, that is to base e. We can get from one base to the other by noting that $\log 10y = \log_e y . \log_{10} e$. To find the value of e on a calculator enter 1 and press exp. $\log_{10}(e)$ is a constant equal to 0.4343. Thus $\log_{10} y = 0.4343 \times \log_e y$.

Try this on a calculator. Put in any positive number and press ln and then exp. You will get back to the original number because $\exp(\ln(x)) = x$.

Note it follows from the definition that for any x, greater than 0, $\log_x(1) = 0$. Try this on a calculator for $\log(1)$ and $\ln(1)$.

In this book exponentials and logarithms feature in a number of places. It is much easier to model data as additive terms in a linear predictor, and yet often terms, such as risk, behave multiplicatively, as discussed in Chapter 3. Taking logs transforms the model from a multiplicative one to an additive one. Logarithms are also commonly used to transform variables which have a positively skewed distribution, because it has been found that this often makes their distribution closer to a Normal distribution. This, of course, won't work if the variable can be zero or negative.

Appendix 2 Maximum likelihood and significance tests

Summary

This appendix gives a brief introduction to the use of *maximum likelihood*, which was the method used to fit the models in the earlier chapters. We describe the *Wald test* and the *likelihood ratio test* and link the latter to the *deviance*. Further details are given in Clayton and Hills.[1]

Binomial models and likelihood

A *model* is a structure for describing data and consists of two parts. The first part describes how the explanatory variables are combined in a linear fashion to give a linear predictor. This is then transformed by a function known as a *link* function to give predicted or fitted values of the outcome variable for an individual. The second part of the model describes the probability distribution of the outcome variable about the predicted value.

Perhaps the simplest model is the Binomial model. An event happens with a probability π. Suppose the event is the probability of giving birth to a boy and suppose we had five expectant mothers who subsequently gave birth to two boys and three girls. The boys were born to mothers numbered 1 and 3. If π is the probability of a boy the probability of this sequence of events occurring is $\pi \times (1-\pi) \times \pi \times (1-\pi) \times (1-\pi)$. If the mothers had different characteristics, say their age, we might wish to distinguish them and write the probability of a boy for mother i as π_i and the probability of a girl as $(1-\pi_i)$ and the probability of the sequence as $\pi_1 \times (1-\pi_2) \times \pi_3 \times (1-\pi_4) \times (1-\pi_5)$. For philosophical and semantic reasons this probability is termed the *likelihood* (in everyday parlance "likelihood" and "probability" are synonyms) for

105

this particular sequence of events and in this case is written $L(\pi)$. The likelihood is the probability of the data, *given* the model.

The process of *maximum likelihood* is to choose the values of π which maximise the likelihood. In Chapter 3 we discussed models for π which are functions of the subject characteristics. For simplicity, here we will consider two extreme cases: the values of π are all the same so we have no information to distinguish individuals, or each π is determined by the data and we can choose each π by whether the outcome is a boy or a girl. In the latter case we can simply choose $\pi_1 = \pi_3 = 1$ and $\pi_2 = \pi_4 = \pi_5 = 0$. This is a *saturated model*, so called because we saturate the model with parameters, and the maximum number possible is to have as many parameters as there are data points (or strictly *degrees of freedom*). In this case

$$L(\pi) = 1 \times (1-0) \times 1 \times (1-0) \times (1-0) = 1$$

If the values of π are all the same, then $L(\pi) = \pi \times (1-\pi) \times \pi \times (1-\pi) \times (1-\pi) = \pi^2 (1-\pi)^3$. In general if there were D boys in N births then $L(\pi) = \pi^D(1-\pi)^{N-D}$. The likelihood, for any particular values of π is a very small number, and it is more convenient to use the natural logarithm of the likelihood instead of the likelihood itself. In this way

$$\log(L(\pi)) = D\log(\pi) + (N-D)\log(1-\pi)$$

It is simple to show that the value of π that maximises the likelihood is the same value that maximises the log-likelihood.

In this expression, the data provide N and D and the statistical problem is to see how $\log(L\pi)$ varies as we vary π, and to choose the value of π that most closely agrees with the data. This is the value of π that maximises $\log(L\pi)$. A graph of the log-likelihood for the data above (two boys and three girls) is given in Figure A2.1.

The maximum occurs at $\pi = 0.4$, which is what one might have guessed. The value at the maximum is given by

$$\log(L(\pi_{max})) = 2\log(0.4) + 3\log(1-0.4) = -3.3651$$

The graph, however is very flat, implying that the maximum is not well estimated. This is because we have very little information with only five observations.

For reasons to be discussed later, the equation for the likelihood

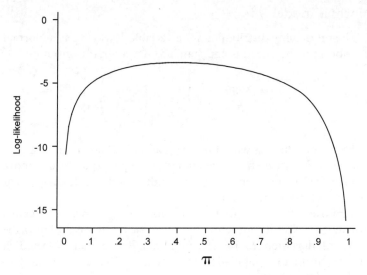

Figure A2.1 Graph of log-likelihood against π, for a Binomial model with D = 2 and N = 5.

is often scaled by the value of the likelihood at the maximum, to give the likelihood ratio, LR(π).

$$LR(\pi)=L(\pi)/L(\pi_{max}) \qquad 0<\pi<1$$

When we take logs(as described in Appendix 1) this becomes

$$\log LR(\pi)=\log\{(L(\pi)\}-\log\{L(\pi_{max})\}$$

Again the maximum occurs when $\pi=0.4$, but in this case the maximum value is zero.

Poisson model

The Poisson model, discussed in Chapter 6, is useful when the number of subjects N is large and the probability of an event, π is small. Then the expected number of events $\lambda=N\pi$ is moderate.

In this case the log likelihood is

$$\log(L(\lambda))=D\log(\lambda)-\lambda$$

Normal model

The probability distribution for a variable Y which has a Normal distribution with mean μ and standard deviation σ is given by

$$\frac{0.3989}{\sigma} \exp\left[\frac{-1}{2}\left(\frac{y-\mu}{\sigma}\right)^2\right]$$

This value changes with differing μ and differing σ. If σ is known (and thus fixed), then this likelihood is simply equal to the above probability but now does not vary with σ and is a function of μ only, which we denote $L(\mu)$.

Suppose we know that adult male height has a Normal distribution. We do not know the mean, $\mu <$ but we do know the standard deviation to be 15 cm. Imagine one man selected at random from this population with height 175cm. Then the log-likelihood of this observation is

$$\log(L(\mu)) = \log(0.3989) - \log(15) - \frac{1}{2}\frac{(175-\mu)^2}{15}$$

The maximum value of $\log L(\mu)$ occurs when $\mu = 175$. This is unsurprising, the single observation is the best estimate of the mean.

The corresponding log-likelihood ratio is given by

$$\text{LogLR}(\mu) = -\frac{1}{2}\frac{(175-\mu)^2}{15} \qquad \text{(A2.1)}$$

This is shown in Figure A.2.2 for different values of μ. Curves with this form are called *quadratic*.

For a series of observations $x_1, x_2, ..., x_n$ we can show that

$$\log LR(\mu) = -\frac{1}{2}\frac{\sum(x_i-\mu)^2}{15}$$

To *maximise* the likelihood we have to *minimise* the sum on the right, because the quantity on the right is negative and small absolute negative values are bigger than large absolute negative

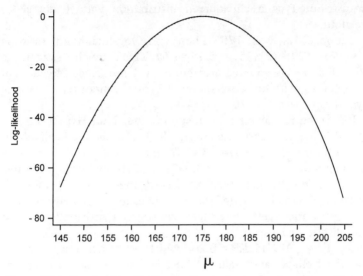

Figure A2.2 Graph of log-likelihood of a single observation from a Normal model.

values (−1 is bigger than −2). Thus we have to choose a value to minimise the sum of squares of the observations from μ. This is the *principle of least squares* described in Chapter 2, and we can see it is equivalent to maximising the likelihood.

Hypothesis testing: likelihood ratio test

Suppose we believed that the true distribution of height for the population from which the man described above was drawn was Normal and had a mean of μ_0. We can put this into equation (A2.1) to calculate the observed log-likelihood ratio.

$$\text{logLR}(\mu_0) = -\frac{1}{2}\frac{(175-\mu_0)^2}{15}$$

Before we can calculate the hypothesis test, we must first use a most useful result for the Normal distribution. The result is that under the Normal distribution,

$$-2 \times (\text{Observed log-likelihood ratio})$$

109

is distributed as a chi-squared distribution with 1 degree of freedom.

Suppose μ_0 was 170. Then $-2 \times$ log-likelihood ratio is $2 \times (175-170)^2/(2 \times 15) = 25/15 = 1.67$. This is much less than the 5% value of a chi-squared distribution with 1 degree of freedom of 3.84 and so, with our observation of 175 we cannot reject the null hypothesis that $\mu_0 = 170$.

Returning to our birth data, suppose our Null Hypothesis was $\pi_0 = 0.5$, i.e. boys and girls are equally likely. The log-likelihood is $2 \times \log(0.5) + 3 \times \log(0.5) = -3.4657$ and the corresponding log-likelihood ratio is $-3.4657 - (-3.3651) = -0.1006$. For non-Normal data the result that $-2 \times$ (Observed log-likelihood ratio) is distributed as a chi-squared distribution is approximately true, and the distribution gets closer to a chi-squared distribution as the sample size increases.

We have $-2 \times \text{logLR} = 0.20$, which is much less than the tabulated chi-squared value of 3.84 and so we cannot reject the null hypothesis. Here the approximation to a chi-squared distribution is likely to be poor because of the small sample size. Intuitively we can see that, because the curve in Figure A2.1 is far from quadratic. However as the sample size increases it will become closer to a quadratic curve.

The log-likelihood is a measure of *goodness-of-fit* of a model. The greater the log-likelihood, the better the fit. Since the absolute value of the log-likelihood is not itself of interest, it is often reported as a log-likelihood ratio compared to some other model. Many computer programs report the *deviance*, which is minus twice the log-likelihood ratio of the model being fitted and a saturated model which includes the maximum number of terms in the model (say as many terms as there are observations). For the birth data above, the saturated model had five parameters, the likelihood was 1 and the log-likelihood 0, and so the deviance in this case is the same as the log-likelihood times minus two. The deviance has degrees of freedom equal to the difference between the number of parameters in the model and the number of parameters in the saturated model.

The deviance is really a measure of badness of fit, not goodness of fit; a large deviance indicates a bad fit. If one model is a subset of another, in that the larger model contains the parameters of the smaller, they can be compared using the differences in their deviances. The change in deviance is minus twice the log-likelihood ratio for the two models because the log-likelihood for the saturated model occurs in both deviances and cancels. The degrees of freedom for this test are found by subtracting the degrees of freedom for the two deviances.

Wald test

When the data are not Normally distributed, the shape of the log-likelihood ratio is no longer quadratic. However, as can be seen from Figure A2.1, it is often approximately so, especially for large samples and there can be advantages in terms of simplicity to using the best quadratic approximation rather than the true likelihood.

Consider a likelihood for a parameter θ of a probability model and let M be the most likely value of θ. A simple quadratic expression is

$$\mathrm{logLR}(\theta) = -\frac{1}{2}\left(\frac{(M-\theta)}{S}\right)^2$$

This has a maximum value of zero when $M = \theta$, and can be used to approximate the true log-likelihood ratio. The parameter S is known as the standard error of the estimate and is used to scale the curve. Small values give sharp peaks of the quadratic curve and large values give flatter peaks. S is chosen to give the closest approximation to the true likelihood *in the region of its most likely value*.

For the binary data given above, with D events out of N the values of M and S are

$$M = D/N$$

and

$$S = \sqrt{\frac{M(1-M)}{N}}$$

For $D = 2$ and $N = 5$ we get $M = 0.4$ and $S = 0.22$.

Under the Null Hypothesis of $\theta = 0.5$, we find that $-2 \times \log LR$ is

$$\left(\frac{(0.4 - 0.5)}{0.22} \right)^2 = 0.21$$

This is close to the log-likelihood ratio value of 0.20 and once again is not statistically significant. This test is commonly used because computer programs obligingly produce estimates of standard errors of parameters. This is equivalent to the z test described in Swinscow[2] of $b/SE(b)$.

Score test

The score test features less often and so we will not describe it in detail. It is based on the gradient of the log-likelihood ratio curve at the null hypothesis. The gradient is often denoted by U and known as the score, evaluated at the null value of the parameter θ_0. Since the slope of a curve at its maximum is zero, if the null hypothesis coincides with the most likely value, then clearly $U = 0$. The score test is based on the fact that under the null hypothesis U^2/V is approximately distributed as a chi-squared distribution with 1 degree of freedom, where V is an estimate of the square of the standard error of the score.

Which method to choose?

For non-Normal data, the methods given above are all approximations. The advantage of the log-likelihood ratio method is that it gives the same P value even if the parameter is transformed (such as by taking logarithms), and so is the generally preferred method. If the three methods give seriously different results it means that the quadratic approximations are not sufficiently close to the true log-likelihood curve in the region going from the null value to the most likely value. This is particularly true if the null value and the most likely value are very far apart, and in this case the choice of the statistical method is most unlikely to affect our scientific conclusions. The Wald test can be improved by a suitable transformation. For example, in a model which includes an odds ratio, reformulating the model for a log odds ratio will improve the quadratic approximation, which is another reason why the log odds ratio is a suitable model in Chapter 3.

All three methods can be generalised to test a number of

parameters simultaneously. However, if one uses a computer program to fit two models, one of which is a subset of the other, then the log-likelihood or the deviance is usually given for each model from which one can derive the log-likelihood ratio for the two models. If the larger model contains two or more parameters more than the smaller model, then the likelihood ratio test of whether the enhanced model significantly improves the fit of the data is a test of all the extra parameters simultaneously.

The parameter estimates and their standard errors are given for each term in a model in a computer output, from which the Wald tests can be derived for each parameter. Thus the simple Wald test tests each parameter separately, not simultaneously with the others. Examples are given in the relevant chapters.

Confidence intervals

The conventional approach to confidence intervals is to use the Wald approach. Thus an approximate 95% confidence interval of a population parameter, for which we have an estimate and a standard error is given by an estimate plus $2 \times SE$ to estimate minus $2 \times SE$. Thus for the birth data an approximate 95% confidence interval is given by $0.6 - 2 \times 0.22$ to $0.6 + 2 \times 0.22 = 0.16$ to 1.04. This immediately shows how poor the approximation is because we cannot have a proportion greater than 1 (for better approximations see Altman *et al*).[3] As in the case of the Wald test, the approximation is improved by a suitable transformation, which is why in Chapter 3 we worked on the log odds ratio, rather than the odds ratio itself. However it is possible to calculate confidence intervals directly from the likelihood which do not require a transformation, and these are occasionally given in the literature. For further details see Clayton and Hills.[1]

References

1 Clayton D, Hills M. *Statistical Models in Epidemiology*. Oxford: OUP, 1993.
2 Swinscrow TDV. *Statistics at Square One, 9th edn* (revised by MJ Campbell). London: BMJ Books, 1996.
3 Altman DG, Machin D, Bryant TN, Gardner MJ, eds. *Statistics with Confidence, 2nd edn*. London: BMJ Books, 2000.

Appendix 3
Bootstrapping

Bootstrapping is a computer-intensive method for estimating parameters and confidence intervals for models that requires fewer assumptions about the distribution of the data than the parametric methods discussed so far. It is becoming much easier to carry out and is available on most modern computer packages.

All the models so far discussed require assumptions concerning the sampling distribution of the estimate of interest. If the sample size is large and we wish to estimate a confidence interval for a mean, then the underlying population distribution is not important because the central limit theorem will ensure that the sampling distribution is approximately Normal. However, if the sample size is small we can only assume a t distribution if the underlying population distribution can be assumed Normal. If this is not the case then the interval cannot be expected to cover the population value with the specified confidence. However, we have information on the distribution of the population from the distribution of the sample data. So-called "bootstrap" estimates (from the expression "pulling oneself up by one's bootstraps") utilise this information, by making repeated random samples of the same size as the original sample from the data, with replacement using a computer. Suitable references are Efron and Tibshirani[1] and Davison and Hinckley.[2]

We seek to mimic in an appropriate manner the way the sample is collected from the population in the bootstrap samples from the observed data. The "with replacement" means that any observation can be sampled more than once. It is important because sampling without replacement would simply give a random permutation of the original data, with many statistics such as the mean being exactly the same. It turns out that "with replacement" is the best way to do this if the observations are independent; if they are not then other methods, beyond the scope of this appendix, are needed. The standard error or confidence interval is estimated from the variability of the statistic derived from the bootstrap samples. The point about the bootstrap is that it produces a variety of values, whose variability reflects the standard error which would be obtained if samples were repeatedly taken from the whole population.

Suppose we wish to calculate a 95% confidence interval for a mean. We take a random sample of the data, of the same size as the original sample, and calculate the mean of the data in this random sample. We do this repeatedly, say 999 times. We now have 999 means. If these are ordered in increasing value a bootstrap 95% confidence interval for the mean would be from the 25th to the 975th values. This is known as the *percentile method* and although it is an obvious choice, it is not the best method of bootstrapping because it can have a bias, which one can estimate and correct for. This leads to methods, such as the *bias corrected method* and the *bias corrected and accelerated (BCa) method*, the latter being the preferred option. There is also the "parametric bootstrap" when the residuals from a *parametric model* are bootstrapped to give estimates of the standard errors of the parameters, for example to estimate the standard errors of coefficients from a multiple regression.

Using the methods above, valid bootstrap P values and confidence intervals can be constructed for all common estimators, such as a proportion, a median, or a difference in means provided the data are independent and come from the same population.

The number of samples required depends on the type of estimator: 50–200 are adequate for a confidence interval for a mean, but 1000 are required for a confidence interval of, say, the 2.5% or 97.5% centiles.

Example

Consider the β-endorphin concentrations from 11 runners described by Dale et al.[3] and also described in Altman et al chapter 13.[4] To calculate a 95% confidence interval for the median using a bootstrap we proceed as follows.

Beta-endorphin concentrations in pmol/l	Median
Original sample: 66, 71.2, 83, 83.6, 101, 107.6, 122, 143, 160, 177, 414	107.6
Bootstrap 1: 143, 107.6, 414, 160, 101, 177, 107.6, 160, 160, 160, 101	160
Bootstrap 2: 122, 414, 101, 83.6, 143, 107.6, 101, 143, 143, 143, 107.6	122
Bootstrap 3: 122, 414, 160, 177, 101, 107.6, 83.6, 177, 177, 107.6, 107.6	122

etc. 999 times

The medians are then ordered by increasing value. The 25th and the 975th values out of 1000 give the percentile estimates of the 95% confidence interval. Using 999 replications we find that the BCa method gives a 95% bootstrap confidence interval 71.2 to 143.0 pmol/l. This contrasts with 71.2 to 177 pmol/l using standard methods given in chapter 5 of Altman *et al.*[4] This suggests that the lower limit for the standard method is probably about right but the upper limit may be too high.

When the standard and the bootstrap methods agree, we can be more confident about the inference we are making and this is an important use of the bootstrap. When they disagree more caution is needed, but the relatively simple assumptions required by the bootstrap method for validity mean that in general it is to be preferred.

It may seem that the best estimator of the median for the population is the median of the bootstrap estimates, but this turns out not to be the case, and the sample median should be quoted as the best estimate of the population median.

The main advantage of the bootstrap is that it frees the investigator from making inappropriate assumptions about the distribution of an estimator in order to make inferences. A particular advantage is that it is available when the formula cannot be derived and it may provide better estimates when the formulae are only approximate.

The so-called "naïve" bootstrap makes the assumption that the sample is an unbiased simple random sample from the study population. More complex sampling schemes, such as stratified random sampling may not be reflected by this, and more complex bootstrapping schemes may be required. Naïve bootstrapping may not be successful in very small samples (say less than nine observations), which are less likely to be representative of the study population. "In very small samples even a badly fitting parametric analysis may outperform a nonparametric analysis, by providing less variable results at the expense of a tolerable amount of bias".[1]

Perhaps one of the most common uses for bootstrapping in medical research has been for calculating confidence intervals for derived statistics such as cost-effectiveness ratios, when the theoretical distribution is mathematically difficult although care is needed here since the denominators in some bootstrap samples can get close to zero.

The bootstrap in action

In health economics, Lambert *et al.*[5] calculated the mean resource costs per patient for day patients with active rheumatoid arthritis as £1789 with a bootstrap 95% confidence interval of £1539 to £2027 (1000 replications).

They used a bootstrap method because the resource costs have a very skewed distribution. However the authors did not state which bootstrap method they used.

Reporting the bootstrap in the literature

* State the method used, such as percentile or bias corrected.

* State the number of replications.

References

1 Efron B and Tibshirani RJ. *An Introduction to the Bootstrap*. New York: Chapman and Hall, 1993.

2 Davison A, Hinckley D. *Bootstrap Methods and their Applications*. Cambridge: Cambridge University Press, 1997.

3 Dale G, Fleetwood JA, Weddell A, Ellis RD, Sainsbury JRC. β-endorphin: a factor in "fun-run"collapse. *BMJ* 1987; **294**: 1004.

4 Altman DG, Machin D, Bryant TN, Gardner MJ, eds *Statistics with Confidence, 2nd edn*. London: BMJ Books, 2000.

5 Lambert CM, Hurst NP, Forbes JF, Lochhead A, Macleod M, Nuki G. Is day care equivalent to inpatient care for active rheumatoid arthritis? Randomised controlled clinical and economic evaluation. *BMJ* 1998; **316**: 965–9.

Appendix 4
Bayesian methods

Consider two clinical trials of equal size for the treatment of headache. One is an analgesic against placebo, and the other is a homoeopathic treatment against placebo. Both give identical P values (<0.05). Which would you believe? The traditional frequentist approach described in the book does not enable one formally to incorporate beliefs about the efficacy of treatment that one might have held before the experiment, but this can be done using *Bayesian methods*.[1]

Bayes' theorem appeared in a posthumous publication in 1763 by Thomas Bayes, a non-conformist minister from Tunbridge Wells. It gives a simple and uncontroversial result in probability theory, relating probabilities of events before an experiment (*a priori*) to probabilities of events after an experiment (*a posteriori*). The link between the prior and the posterior is the *likelihood*, described in Appendix 2. Specific uses of the theorem have been the subject of considerable controversy for many years and it is only in recent years a more balanced and pragmatic perspective has emerged.[2]

A familiar situation to which Bayes' theorem can be applied is diagnostic testing; a doctor's prior belief about whether a patient has a particular disease (based on knowledge of the prevalence of the disease in the community and the patient's symptoms) will be modified by the result of the test.[3] Bayesian methods enable one to make statements such as "the probability that the new treatment is better than the old is 0.95". Under certain circumstances, 95% confidence intervals calculated in the conventional (frequentist) manner can be interpreted as "a range of values within which one is 95% certain that the true value of a parameter really lies".[4] Thus it can be argued that a Bayesian approach allows results to be presented in a form that is most suitable for decisions. Bayesian methods interpret data from a study in the light of external evidence and judgement, and the form in which conclusions are drawn contributes naturally to decision-making.[5] Prior plausibility of hypotheses is taken into account, just as when interpreting the results of a diagnostic test. Scepticism about large treatment effects can be formally expressed and used in cautious interpretation of results that cause surprise.

One of the main difficulties with Bayesian methods is the choice of the prior distribution. Different analysts may choose different priors, and so the same data set analysed by different investigators could lead to different conclusions. A commonly chosen prior is an *uninformative prior,* which assigns equal probability to all values over the possible range and leads to analyses that are possibly less subjective than analyses that use priors based on, say, clinical judgement. There are philosophical differences between Bayesians and frequentists, such as the nature of probability, but these should not interfere with a sensible interpretation of data.

A Bayesian perspective leads to an approach to clinical trials that is claimed to be more flexible and ethical than traditional methods.[6]

Bayesian methods do not supplant traditional methods, but complement them. In this book the area of greatest overlap would be in random effects models, described in Chapter 5. Further details are given by Berry and Stangl.[7]

Reporting Bayesian methods in the literature[8]

- Report the pre-experiment probabilities and specify how they were determined. In most practical situations, the particular form of the prior information has little influence on the final outcome because it is overwhelmed by the weight of experimental evidence.

- Report the post-trial probabilities and their intervals. Often the mode of the posterior distribution is reported, with the 2.5 and 97.5 centiles (the 95% prediction interval). It can be helpful to plot the posterior distribution.

References

1 Bland JM, Altman DG. Bayesians and frequentists. *BMJ* 1998; **317**: 1151–2.
2 Spiegelhalter DJ, Myles JP, Jones DR, Abrams KR. Methods in health service research: an introduction to Bayesian methods in health technology assessment. *BMJ* 1999; **319**: 508–12.
3 Campbell MJ, Machin D. *Medical Statistics: A commonsense approach, 3rd edn.* Chichester: John Wiley, 1999.
4 Burton PR, Gurrin LC, Campbell MJ. Clinical significance not statistical significance: a simple Bayesian alternative to P values. *J Epidemiol Community Health* 1998; **52**: 318–23.
5 Lilford RJ, Braunholtz D. The statistical basis of public policy: a paradigm shift is overdue. *BMJ* 1996; **313**: 603–7.
6 Kadane JB. Prime time for Bayes. *Control Clin Trials* 1995; **16**: 313–18.
7 Berry DA, Stangl DK. *Bayesian Biostatistics.* New York: Marcel Dekker, 1996.
8 Hughes MD. Reporting Bayesian analyses of clinical trials. *Statist in Med* 1993; **12**: 1651–63, .

Answers to exercises

Chapter 1

1. Types of data.
   (i) Categorical, (ii) Continuous (non-Normal), (iii) Categorical, (iv) Ordinal, (v) Continuous, (vi) Continuous, (vii) Binary, (viii) Discrete quantitative.

2. Casual/confounder/outcome variables.
   (i) True, (ii) False (there are two types of diet and they are causal), (iii) True, (iv) True, (v) False: it is a binary variable.

3. Basic statistics.
   (i) False. Despite being non-significant, the CI value is large. (ii) True. (iii) True. (iv) False. There is a 45% chance of getting the observed difference or one more extreme if CBT and drug treatment were the same. (v) False. A new trial is likely to have a CI that overlaps the old, but the mean difference for a new trial is not the population mean.

Chapter 2

1. (i)False. It is the residuals having allowed for median share of income, median income and country that is assumed normal. (ii)True ($330 = 282 + 53 - 5$). (iii)False. It is the relationship between median *share* that is assumed different. (iv)True. (v)True.

2. (i)False. X_1 and X_2 can be discrete. (ii)False. It depends on X_1 and X_2. (iii)False. Changing values of X_1 will alter relationship with X_2 and so affect b_2. (iv)True. (v)True.

Chapter 3

1. (i) False (the confidence interval includes 1). (ii) True. (iii) False. The study is unmatched. (iv) True. (v) True.

2. (i) True. (ii) True. (iii) True. (iv) False (see discussion of conditional logistic regression). (v) False. If the matching factors are of no prognostic value, conditional and unconditional analyses may agree quite closely.

Chapter 4

A = 3 (three parameters in model). B = 1.10 ($-2\times(188.55165-188.04719)$). C = -0.487 ($=-0.1512/0.3102$). Note: It is *not* the ratio of the hazard ratio to its standard error. 0.626. D = -0.7592 ($=-0.1512-1.96\times0.3102$) E = 0.4568 ($=-0.1512+1.96\times0.3102$). F = 0.4680 ($=\exp(-0.7592)$). G = 1.5790 ($=\exp(0.4568)$).

1. Likelihood ratio = 10.71 ($=-2\times(188.0472-182.6898)$). DF = 4 (four dummy variables).
2. 0.763 (95% CI -0.272 to 2.136).
3. $(0.9978)^{10} = 0.9782$.

Index